Trauma & Young Children

Teaching Strategies to Support & Empower

Sarah Erdman & Laura J. Colker
with Elizabeth C. Winter

The National Association for the Education of Young Children
Washington, DC

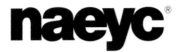

National Association for the
Education of Young Children
1313 L Street NW, Suite 500
Washington, DC 20005-4101
202-232-8777 • 800-424-2460
NAEYC.org

NAEYC Books

Senior Director, Publishing
and Professional Learning
Susan Friedman

Director, Books
Dana Battaglia

Senior Editor
Holly Bohart

Editor
Rossella Procopio

Senior Creative Design Manager
Henrique J. Siblesz

Senior Creative Design Specialist
Charity Coleman

Senior Creative Design Specialist
Gillian Frank

Publishing Business
Operations Manager
Francine Markowitz

Through its publications program,
the National Association
for the Education of Young
Children (NAEYC) provides a
forum for discussion of major
issues and ideas in the early
childhood field, with the hope
of provoking thought and
promoting professional growth.
The views expressed or implied
in this book are not necessarily
those of the Association.

Contents

Preface

This book was headed to the printer as the novel coronavirus (COVID-19) was taking a firm hold on the United States and around the world. A global pandemic reaches every community, although the impact is different for each person. There are people directly affected by the illness or death of loved ones; the economic impacts of job and wage loss; increased stress and anxiety, magnified for many people by isolation; and the loss of familiarity, structure, and routine. For some, this may have been the first real crisis they have experienced; for others, it may trigger past trauma. For everyone, there is the fear of the unknown. Some psychologists have labeled the anxiety that engulfs us all as grief (Berinato 2020). And like any type of grief, it has to be dealt with and processed in the same way that trauma is.

The needs at the time of this writing, while the pandemic is still spreading and unmanaged, are different than they will be in the months, years, and decades afterward. However, this event will leave its mark on a generation of children both in the immediate future and as those children grow up. Many people have compared the pandemic to the 9/11 terrorist attacks in the United States, illustrating how one event forever changes the course of our lives.

Our sense of safety and security, whatever that looked like before the pandemic, has been taken from us, leaving us feeling fragile and uncertain. The stresses of living in close quarters without outside support and the economic strain of lost wages create an environment ripe for adverse childhood experiences, or ACEs (discussed in detail in this book), and leave children and families vulnerable to other traumas.

The closing or limiting of participation in schools, child care centers, and family child care programs has interrupted the relationships with children and families that so many educators have labored hard to develop. It will take more hard work and perhaps novel approaches to reestablish these connections and help children work through their fears, both those related to the pandemic and those they may have been grappling with previously.

Although COVID-19 has dominated the news cycle for months, the conversation and coverage will change as the situation develops and stabilizes. Even after the pandemic is no longer headline news, it will linger as a potential source of trauma and children and adults will be processing the experience and effects in their own ways throughout their lives. This is true for other current events as well, like families separated at the southern border of the United States; communities grappling with gun violence; and citizens, cities, and countries battling the effects of climate change.

While the aftereffects of this pandemic are unknown at this time, there is a stronger need than ever to work to help mitigate the negative effects of trauma on children. Collectively, we must turn fears into positivity and work proactively to support children, families, and ourselves. We hope this book serves as a multipurpose tool in your kit of resources. Instead of feeling buffeted by the changes in the world around you, whatever they are, you can use your knowledge of how children grow and develop along with the strategies presented in this book and other resources to support children, their families, your education community, and yourself. More than ever, informed, compassionate, and high-quality early childhood educators are critical to the framework of society. We are grateful for the work you put in and your drive to continue to learn and improve for the good of the communities you serve. You are on the front line of giving meaning to a frightening time in history. The hope and assistance you offer children and families will enable children to go forward and flourish.

—Sarah Erdman and Laura J. Colker
April 2020

There is a reason you picked up this book. Maybe you are worried about a child in your care, either because you know something is happening with the child and family or because you feel like there is more than what you can see. Maybe you see a pattern in your program or community of children who are exposed to stressful or dangerous situations and you want to make broad changes that will address these situations. Or perhaps it is because of the regular and repeated media reports of gun violence, natural disasters, global pandemics, and refugee and migrant children being separated from their families. Early childhood educators are bombarded with the reality of trauma in young children's lives, and the information in this book is a definitive step toward making a difference. Not only do you see the issue and want to make change, but you are also finding the resources to make it happen.

Why It Is Important to Understand Trauma

Young children need guidance and support to thrive emotionally, socially, cognitively, linguistically, and physically. For many children, trauma disrupts this development, making it challenging to learn until the effects are addressed. It is critical that early childhood educators be able to support children and help them develop resilience and coping strategies. Nearly every educator will interact with a child or family who has been affected by trauma, and research shows that the support and intervention a child receives when young can make a critical difference.

Most educators, however, have not been trained in appropriate practices for addressing traumatic response in young children. Indeed, you may even be unclear about what trauma is or whether what you are seeing in the children in your program is characterized as traumatic response. It is even more unclear how you should respond to these experiences. In addition, you or your colleagues may have experienced trauma and may be dealing with its ongoing effects.

In this seemingly unstable world, it is easy to feel hopeless and overwhelmed. However, educators can have an immediate and lasting impact on children who experience trauma because of their understanding of how children grow and develop and the opportunity they have to build strong relationships with children. With knowledge, resources, and support to react appropriately and wisely, you can take steps that will turn a seemingly depressing situation into a hopeful outcome.

Supporting children who have experienced trauma guides your choices in what the learning environment looks like, how you respond to children, what skills you focus on, and your interactions with families. Understanding the science behind trauma and traumatic response, what trauma does to the brain, and the different types of trauma and triggers also gives you insight into children's behaviors.

This book gives educators of children in preschool and kindergarten programs information about trauma, what it is, how it occurs, and what its effects might look like in children's behavior. It also offers strategies that support all children's social and emotional well-being and their learning. This information can inform a preservice teacher or new educator's practice, and it can help experienced educators, directors, and trainers adapt what they already do to include new

All Early Childhood Educators Are Professionals

All educators who work with children and their families are professionals. In this book we refer to all of those professionals—whether they work in center-based programs, public or private schools, family child care programs, or other early learning settings—as *educators* or *teachers*.

research and understanding. Young children *can* work through the effects of trauma. And with your help and appropriate supports from your program and community, they can even flourish.

Prevalence of Trauma

Trauma comes in many forms, and its effects can manifest in dramatically different ways depending on the child. Trauma occurs when a child witnesses or experiences an event that is a threat (real or perceived) to themselves or someone close to them. Traumatic events can range from dealing with a threatening hurricane or the lingering effects of a global pandemic to experiencing abuse to losing a loved one. Trauma can overwhelm the child's ability to cope and cause a chain reaction of feelings like fear and hopelessness as well as changes in behavior or health (Nicholson, Perez, & Kurtz 2019). Outside factors, such as the support system a child has or their previous experiences with trauma, play a huge part in how children respond and recover.

One out of every four children attending school has been exposed to a traumatic event that can affect learning and behavior (National Child Traumatic Stress Network [NCTSN] 2008a). Trauma doesn't just happen to older children and teens; research shows that 26 percent of children in the United States will have witnessed or experienced trauma before the age of 4 (Statman-Weil 2015). Children of any gender or age and from every type of family, socioeconomic background, culture, and geographic region experience trauma. But while trauma can happen to any child, the prevalence is not evenly distributed across populations. Certain communities are disproportionately affected by trauma because of generations of discrimination and lack of access to support systems, and other groups face specific types of trauma in higher numbers. Chapter 2 provides more discussion on these topics.

Trauma-Informed Care

Trauma-informed care (TIC) is a term prevalent in education, juvenile justice departments, mental health programs, and youth development agencies. TIC can be defined as a strengths-based service delivery approach "grounded in an understanding of and responsiveness to the impact of trauma; that emphasizes physical, psychological, and emotional safety for both teachers and survivors; that creates opportunities for survivors to rebuild a sense of control and empowerment" (Hopper, Bassuk, & Olivet 2010, 82). The ultimate goal of TIC is that children who have experienced trauma can heal and learn to thrive.

At its core, TIC "encourages support and treatment to the whole person, rather than focusing on only treating individual symptoms or specific behaviors" (Ginwright 2018). TIC also reinforces the idea that trauma does not define a child. Rather than looking at behaviors as problems that need to be solved, TIC urges looking at the source of behavior and what steps can be used to help ease it. It also emphasizes that the details of a child's trauma are not what is important; what is critical is looking at how to care for the whole person. Experts such as Shawn Ginwright and Ellen Galinsky emphasize the need for a wellness and strengths-based approach that focuses on healing-centered engagement for children who have been exposed to trauma.

Singular Pronouns in this Book

Throughout this book we use the singular *they*, *them*, and *theirs* when referring to someone who uses those pronouns or whose pronouns are not explicitly stated and when the use of gender-based pronouns isn't critical to the context. This is a growing and encouraged practice to reduce bias. It not only breaks down stereotypes about gender (for example, that all early childhood teachers use *she*) but also reaffirms that all readers are part of the narrative.

The term *TIC* can be an important reminder to educators. Just as your teaching philosophy, curriculum, and day-to-day interactions are informed by what you know about child development and the needs of the children and their families and communities, these aspects should also be informed by a better understanding of the role trauma can play in children's lives. Throughout the book, remember that TIC does not mean seeing a child only through the lens of the trauma they have experienced. Rather, it is a is healing-centered and strengths-based approach.

Early Childhood Educators Matter

Children who have experienced trauma may believe that the world is a scary, threatening place. They may exhibit challenging behavior or have less developed social and emotional skills that make it difficult for them to regulate their emotions and be successful in interactions with their peers and adults. Their cognitive skills and physical development may also be negatively affected by trauma.

Educators like you are a critical resource for children who have experienced trauma. Not only do you build a close relationship with the child and their family, you also can provide targeted, developmentally appropriate support through the learning environment you create and the choices you make in how you interact with children and families. By creating a safe environment and nurturing positive relationships, you help build up children's strengths and provide them with opportunities for success.

Family dynamics play a role in many causes of trauma and affect how the child responds and develops resilience. Supporting families is a significant part of helping children cope with trauma. Working with family members, your colleagues, and your community will help you build a wide network of support for families.

The most important piece of TIC is you. Continuing to learn and improve your practice is vital, but so is understanding your own experience with trauma and how to continue being responsive without burning out. Self-care is critical to balancing the needs of children and families with your own physical and mental health and is discussed in Chapter 10.

A Path Forward

Trauma in young children is a crisis, and as is true for other types of crises, it takes a network of individuals and organizations to provide support and make real change. While you cannot solve the needs of the children you work with alone, your voice and effort are critical components. Learning how to use healing-centered practices and focusing on supporting children's strengths is incredibly helpful in both the short and long term. By educating yourself about trauma and how it can affect children and taking steps to make your program and practice responsive to the needs of children and families, you will add to the network and make a more effective safety net for children and families.

The overarching goal of this book is to provide you with support as you interact with children and families. Each chapter describes current research and best practices and offers specific strategies or suggestions. The appendices provide additional resources for learning and application, including print and digital resources, suggested picture books, and handouts for families. This book is one among many resources at your disposal; numerous organizations provide information and trainings for professionals, families, schools, and communities.

We hope this book serves as a scaffold or stepladder, giving you relevant information on useful strategies to build your understanding of trauma and traumatic response in children and the role you can play in helping them not only survive but flourish.

CHAPTER
Two

Types of Trauma Experienced by Young Children

Early childhood educators are constantly adjusting their practice to meet children where they are and help them reach challenging and achievable goals—core tenets of developmentally appropriate practice (DAP) (Copple & Bredekamp 2009). To provide a learning environment for children that embraces excellence and equity, teachers incorporate a thorough understanding of how children develop and learn, how to teach based on children's unique characteristics and experiences, and what each child's social, family, and cultural contexts mean for learning (NAEYC 2009; NAEYC 2019). This concept is critical; children don't fit neatly into specific boxes, with one approach covering everyone's needs.

This same mindset applies when you are striving to be aware of and sensitive to the needs of children who have experienced trauma and their families. Even knowing that a child has been in a traumatic circumstance, because you observed it firsthand or were told by a reliable source who has a relationship with the child, doesn't give you the full picture or tell you what strategies would best support the child and family.

In addition, if you aren't told directly about the circumstances, it is easy to fall into the trap of relying on guesswork, unconscious bias, a child's behavior, and your own experience to assume that a particular child has experienced a traumatic situation. However, all of these can lead you to unfounded conclusions. Educating yourself on what trauma is, understanding potential sources, and learning what a traumatic response may look like in a child enables you to better recognize a child who needs support in the moment and partner with the family to find ways to ease the causes of the trauma. This lets you better individualize your response and care for the whole child rather than trying to address individual behaviors.

This chapter explores broad definitions of trauma and then looks more closely at different types and the presentation you may see in a child who has been exposed to that type of trauma. It is critical to keep in mind, as Ellen Galinsky notes, that "adversity is not destiny" and that a caring person can have an enormous impact on a child's life ("From Trauma-Informed to Asset-Informed Care in Early Childhood," Brookings, October 23, 2018). Later chapters will speak about effective strategies that you can use as you build relationships and provide healing-centered TIC in your environment.

What Is Trauma?

Trauma is defined as "an experience that threatens life or physical integrity and overwhelms the capacity to cope" (NCTSN 2008b). There are two major categories of trauma: acute and complex. *Acute trauma* is "a single exposure to an overwhelming event" (Sorrels 2015), such as being involved in a car crash or experiencing an extreme weather event like a flood or tornado. It can also come from witnessing a violent incident.

Unlike acute trauma, complex trauma is not a one-time event. *Complex trauma* refers to chronic and ongoing harm or neglect at the hands of another, with far-reaching, long-term effects (see NCTSN, n.d. b). It also refers to trauma that occurs within a more finite period of time but has effects that linger, like extensive recovery from an injury or serious illness that leaves a child with trauma related to medical procedures. In young children, complex trauma usually happens within a family or caregiver relationship, because children are completely dependent on others to care for them. Complex trauma includes all forms of abuse (physical, emotional, sexual), neglect, and abandonment as well as living in an environment with domestic violence (Sorrels 2015).

Trauma can be experienced in different ways. Firsthand trauma refers to events that happen to a child or to the child's family member in a way that directly influences the child's experience. This could be an acute traumatic event or a complex, ongoing trauma.

Secondhand trauma, sometimes called *secondary trauma*, is defined by "indirect exposure to trauma through a firsthand account or narrative of a traumatic event" (Zimering & Gulliver 2003). A child might experience secondhand trauma through watching news footage of a terrorist attack, hearing about community violence from adults, or having a close, trusted adult who has experienced trauma. Although the child does not experience the trauma themselves, hearing the vivid recounting or seeing images of traumatic events can deeply affect them because of the connection they feel to adults closest to them and their perception of time, which may make them think that the event is happening at that moment.

People who work closely with children, including educators, social workers, and therapists, can also experience secondhand trauma. These professionals may find that their work takes an emotional toll and that they begin to have symptoms that parallel post-traumatic stress disorder (PTSD). In these scenarios, secondhand trauma is sometimes called *compassion fatigue* or *vicarious trauma*. This type of trauma is discussed in more depth in Chapter 10.

Key Concepts Related to Trauma

There are three key concepts to keep in mind when thinking about trauma and young children. The first is that *the way an individual experiences trauma is completely dependent on that person's perspective*, no matter how an outside person views the experience.

Second, *trauma is not only the event itself but the response to the stressful situation and the undermining of the person's ability to manage.* While a specific event may be the catalyst, what comes after is also significant. The emphasis on relationship-based and healing-centered approaches in early childhood programs is in direct response to this idea.

Third, *trauma and its impact are subjective; a child's worldview and previous experiences will determine how they interpret and respond to the event.* For one child, having a parent who is

hospitalized may be distressing while it is happening but not affect them long term. However, a different child may experience lasting negative effects from a similar event.

Adverse Childhood Experiences

Discussions of trauma often include the mention of adverse childhood experiences (ACEs)—potentially traumatic events that occur in childhood. This term comes from a landmark study conducted by the Centers for Disease Control and Prevention (CDC) and Kaiser Permanente from 1995 to 1997 that measured ten types of childhood trauma (Felitti et al. 1998). Individuals participating in the study marked the adverse experiences they had been exposed to as children, which were then tallied to give them an overall ACE score. The childhood traumas listed included five personally experienced traumas and five involving family members:

> Physical abuse

> Verbal abuse

> Sexual abuse

> Physical neglect

> Emotional neglect

> A family member who was a substance abuser

> A mother who was a victim of domestic violence

> A family member who was incarcerated

> A family member with a severe mental illness

> Parents who were separated or divorced

Researchers found that a higher ACE score put individuals at increased risk for later negative outcomes in health and well-being, including mental illness, risky behaviors such as substance use disorders, and diminished professional and educational opportunities (Sacks & Murphey 2018). Nationally, 1 in 10 children have experienced three or more ACEs and just under half of all children in the United States have experienced at least one ACE (Sacks & Murphey 2018).

Causes of Trauma

Understanding potential sources of trauma in a child's life helps you keep in mind the big picture of how home, family, and community have an impact on a child's response to traumatic events. It also allows you to access support strategies more quickly and to individualize them. The ACE study (Felitti et al. 1998) greatly helped shape discussion of potential traumatic events. However, as the knowledge of trauma and trauma-informed care has progressed, the understanding of what constitutes an adverse experience has also developed. Noting that the "body's stress response does not distinguish between overt threats from inside or outside the home environment, it just recognizes when there *is* a threat, and goes on high alert," the National Scientific Council on the Developing Child "expanded its definition of adversity beyond the categories that were the focus of the initial ACE study to include community and systemic causes—such as violence in the child's community and experiences with racism and chronic poverty" (Center on the Developing Child, n.d. a).

With that in mind, potential traumas are discussed here within four broad categories.

> **Household and family:** Trauma that arises from within a child's household, family, or primary care situations, including physical, emotional, and sexual abuse; neglect; severe or chronic illness; family discord; and financial insecurity and poverty

> **Loss:** Reactions to death experienced by a child, including the loss of someone important to the child and traumatic grief

> **Family separation:** Trauma that occurs when a child is separated from their family or a particular family member; includes situations in which families are refugees or migrants or a family member is incarcerated or deployed

> **Violence and disaster:** Violent events that affect children, including gun violence, natural and human-made disasters, car crashes, personal injury and witnessing violence, and terrorism

Category 1: Household and Family

Young children are dependent on their family for their physical and emotional safety; thus, it is more likely that complex trauma will arise from within the household. However, there are many ways this can manifest.

Physical Abuse

Physical abuse is committing an act that results in physical injury to the child, including bruises, burns, and broken bones.

Physical abuse from a parent or guardian is especially toxic because a child's natural instinct is to run *to* that person for protection, but when abuse is occurring, their stress response will tell them to run *away* instead (Sorrels 2015). This leaves the child with no clear person to turn to and keeps them in a heightened state of fear and alarm.

Physical abuse may have many lasting behavioral effects. Children may have difficulty forming relationships, because they learned early on not to trust anyone or to default to aggression to solve conflict. They also can feel like they deserved the abuse and have a sense of worthlessness. Some children show hypervigilance—being abnormally alert to the potential of danger and threat, demonstrating increased aggression or instances of acting out, and experiencing a constant state of alarm. Hypervigilance may also be related to a higher incidence of ADD and ADHD diagnosis among children experiencing trauma, because the symptoms are similar (Sorrels 2015). Later in this chapter there is further discussion of misdiagnoses that often occur.

Children who experience physical abuse also may turn to risky behaviors or substance use disorders later in life as a means of coping. If you suspect physical abuse or any other type of abuse discussed below, you must follow your state's reporting requirements immediately.

Emotional Abuse

Emotional abuse does not have a single, accepted definition, and it can be difficult to detect. It is characterized by behaviors that are meant to diminish someone's feelings of dignity, confidence, and self-worth. It may be inflicted by family members intentionally taunting or humiliating a child or creating a climate in which the child feels frightened. Children can also experience emotional abuse when they feel overpressured or isolated from normal social experiences.

Children who have experienced emotional abuse may develop a paralyzing sense of shame and humiliation, seeing themselves as unworthy of love or affection and trying to remain unnoticed. They may be developmentally delayed or show physical manifestations such as frequent stomachaches or headaches and fluctuating weight. Socially, they may have difficulty forming relationships or be aggressive and cruel or withdrawn. They may also demonstrate behaviors that seem inappropriate for their age, such as an older child continuing to suck their thumb or rock their body.

Sexual Abuse

Sexual abuse is when a child is used for another person's sexual stimulation. It can happen between a child and an adult or between a child and another child. Sexual abuse can include witnessing sexual activity or pornography or being used for sexual exploitation for pornographic purposes as well as inappropriate bodily contact like fondling, kissing, or intercourse (Sorrels 2015).

Children who have experienced sexual abuse may have no personal boundaries and initiate or accept inappropriate bodily contact. They may also have sexual knowledge, behaviors, or language beyond their age. In addition, they may experience behavior changes like being depressed and withdrawn or having angry outbursts. Their sleep may be affected or they may express fear of being left alone with particular individuals. Educators may also observe a child re-enacting the experience through play or talking about their body as being hurt or dirty (NCTSN, n.d. c).

Neglect

Neglect is defined by an inadequate response to a child's needs. This can include lack of basic survival needs like access to food, shelter, and medical care; lack of supervision; and lack of experiences or sensory stimulations.

A child who is neglected may develop medical problems like malnutrition and chronic physical pain as well as headaches or stomachaches. Children who are neglected may also have an over- or undersensitivity to pain, touch, smells, sounds, and light.

Beyond the risks to a child's physical health, neglect carries risks for learning deficits and language and other developmental delays; the constant stress on a child's body and brain from neglect affects growth and development. Neglected children may have difficulty forming relationships, and there may be an increase in anxiety or other mental health issues. Emotional responses can be unpredictable and explosive.

Identifying neglect can be difficult. A child may seem constantly tired, hungry, unclean, or not dressed appropriately for the weather. They may need medical care or be frequently absent from the program. The child may also make comments about no one being home to provide care. In addition, the parent may seem apathetic or indifferent to the child or be depressed or irrational.

Family Dysfunction and Household Instability

Other sources of instability in a child's life may contribute to adverse experiences. A family member with mental health issues may exhibit abusive or neglectful behaviors, or their interactions may create a chaotic and unpredictable household environment. As explained at the beginning of this chapter, trauma occurs not only when life and physical integrity are threatened but also when an individual's capacity to cope is overwhelmed (Sorrels 2015). Baseline chaos in a child's home, like not knowing who will be there to care for them or having irregular meals or disrupted schedules, diminishes a child's resilience and capacity for response when traumatic events occur on top of what the child is already trying to manage.

Severe and Chronic Illness

Children thrive on predictability and routines, and having a family member with a chronic or severe illness, even if it is generally well managed, can make their life feel erratic. Often the people who serve as the caregiver for the ill individual are worried and anxious and may be taking on different roles and responsibilities in the family. There might be changes in the family's financial situation or daily routine. Disruptions for medical procedures, times when the ill person is unavailable to the child, or sudden changes in the health of the person can create uncertainty and concern.

If a child is the one who is ill, then they are dealing with all of the unpredictability, uncertainty, and anxiety related to disruption of routine as well as the physical symptoms of their illness. Invasive medical procedures can spark lifelong anxiety and medical trauma. Very young children do not understand that the pain, surgeries, needles, or tubes are lifesaving; their bodies and brains interpret the situations as the people around them causing them pain (Sorrels 2015). Children react to how frightening the event is for them rather than responding objectively to the severity of the problem.

Family Discord

Family discord is a general term for anything that creates instability and uncertainty in a household. This can include, but is not limited to, substance use disorders, substance use happening in the home, family members experiencing severe mental illness, or family members thinking about or planning suicide.

Family discord can affect social development and make it difficult for children to form relationships. It is not only a risk for trauma in its own right, but it can also lead to other types of abuse or neglect if it is not addressed. Children may have insufficient supervision or lack stimulation. Their basic needs may not be taken care of or the family member may be physically abusive.

Children living with family discord may show a variety of symptoms, such as hypervigilance, withdrawal, or anxiety and clinging behavior with trusted adults. Some children take on caregiving roles or try to constantly be a peacemaker.

Financial Insecurity and Poverty

Nearly 1 in 5 children in the United States—12.8 million in total—live in poverty, which at the time of this writing is defined as having an annual family income of less than $25,000 a year for a family of four (Children's Defense Fund 2019). While poverty isn't an automatic catalyst for trauma in children, it is considered by some to be a source of trauma on its own (Menschner & Maul 2016) and often causes conditions that factor into other sources of trauma.

Families who are living at or below the poverty line can experience extreme stress because of tight budgets and the disparities between income and cost of living. They may lack necessities like food, safe housing, and health care and live in areas with environmental hazards, a lack of safe play spaces, and increased violence. Children's education may be interrupted frequently or of low quality. For some families, the stressors may lead to abuse, neglect, and other types of trauma.

Children living in low-income communities face significantly more ACEs and environmental risk factors than children from higher-income families: 13 percent of children living at or below the poverty line have had three or more ACEs, compared with 5 percent of children in households with income more than twice the poverty level (Child Trends 2019). It is estimated that 50 to 80 percent of children living in poverty have experienced trauma (NEA 2016). In addition, children in poverty are less likely to overcome these traumas because there is rarely a break in their exposure to ongoing ACEs and other types of trauma (Collins et al. 2010). Children of color are significantly more likely to be poor compared with White children (Children's Defense Fund 2019; Jensen 2016) and thus are disproportionately affected by poverty-related traumas.

Many children living in these conditions of instability and upheaval experience chronic or toxic stress, which is long-term stress that has been linked to physical and developmental delays (see Chapter 3 for more on toxic stress). The hormone cortisol and other stress markers are continually elevated—a sign of toxic stress—in children who live in poverty (Blair & Raver 2016), and this can cause changes in brain architecture.

These changes adversely affect executive function and emotional regulation, which in turn impacts children's ability to thrive in school (Blair & Raver 2016).

Poverty does not automatically mean a child will experience long-term effects from trauma, however. Many families can draw on cultural and spiritual resources to provide a buffer from the adverse effects of trauma (Christian & Barbarin 2001; NCTSN, n.d. a; Wethington et al. 2008). And educators, as discussed in Chapter 4, play an important role in mitigating these effects.

Category 2: Loss

Being confronted with death is an experience that almost every child will have in one form or another. Whether it is a loved one or family pet or even seeing a dead insect or bird, being able to cope with these upsets is foundational to children's emotional and mental health. Death can happen suddenly or be a planned-for transition. There may also be outside influences like long illness or substance use that affect how children and the adults in their life cope with death. In addition, the myriad personal, societal, and cultural norms surrounding death influence how it is experienced by the child and the process they learn for dealing with it. Trusted adults are critical in helping children process what has happened and guiding them through healthy ways to cope.

Loss of Someone Important to the Child

Although any death may affect a child, the loss of someone important to them will bring up a complex array of emotions. They may feel anger and confusion along with their grief, and depending on their age and developmental level, they will have an evolving understanding of what death means. Preschool-aged children may also think their actions have the power to change reality and if they thought or said bad things about a person, it might have caused that person to die.

Traumatic Grief

In many cases, children can grieve a loss while still maintaining routines and achieving developmental milestones. Sometimes, though, a child will develop what the NCTSN refers to as a "traumatic grief response" (NCTSN, n.d. d), which occurs when they are unable to cope with the changes that resulted from the death and move forward with healthy patterns of living. Traumatic grief response usually occurs following the loss of a primary attachment figure (such as a parent or sibling) or another important person in the child's life, such as a relative, friend, or classmate (NCTSN, n.d. d).

Children who are experiencing traumatic grief may

> Withdraw and avoid any reminders or triggers of the loss

> Experience distress when reminded of the person—even of happy times

> Be irritable and angry

> Complain of headaches or stomachaches

> Be overly vigilant about their safety and the safety of others

> Have guilt or blame themselves for the death of the person

> Have nightmares (NCTSN, n.d. d)

In most cases, children who are experiencing traumatic grief require intervention from a mental health professional to help them work through the grief and learn to cope.

Category 3: Family Separation

For young children, who rely entirely on their families to take care of them, family separations can be incredibly traumatizing. Children may experience separation in a number of ways.

Refugees and Migrants

Children who leave their country of origin with their families as refugees or migrants experience a variety of events that may be traumatic. They may have witnessed violence and war, including torture and assault, or may have lost loved ones. They also may have lacked necessities like food and shelter or been injured and ill and had their schooling disrupted. Often, they have left familiar surroundings and family and friends.

Hardships may continue after arriving in a new country, including the difficulties of making a new life and building a community of support and resources. Children often pick up on the anxiety and stress of their family members. They may have difficulty fitting in at school or in their family child care program. For young children who are learning to speak both English and their home language, known as dual language learners, the burdens of trauma become heavier than they might ordinarily be if children can't communicate effectively with the people around them (K. Nemeth, personal communication). If educators do not speak the home languages of the children in their care, the ability to form a strong bond is weakened at a time when children need to connect the most.

Children who are refugees also risk being separated from their families and communities. For young children, who build their entire identity on the people in their lives who take care of them, losing their main ties to their family and community makes them vulnerable to trauma and traumatic response.

For the estimated 1 million undocumented immigrant children living in the United States (APA, n.d.), this status predisposes them to open-ended stress. In addition to the traumas they likely experienced in their country of origin or at the border, they may experience the possibility of immigration raids in their communities, arbitrary stopping of family members to check their documentation status, and the threat of deportation.

Any of these stressors may have a strong impact on a child, and when multiple stressors are layered on top of each other, as is often the case with refugee and migrant children, it can affect a child's physical and mental health, including difficulty eating and sleeping, withdrawal, and anxiety (APA, n.d.). A growing awareness of the potential for these stressors and more resources being shared among educators and other professionals means that the circumstances of refugee and migrant children are being recognized, with the goal of specific supports being put in place.

Incarceration

Over 1.5 million children in the United States have at least one parent incarcerated. Black children are overwhelmingly affected: 1 out of 9 have an incarcerated parent, compared with 1 in 28 Latino children and 1 in 57 White children (National Resource Center on Children & Families of the Incarcerated 2014). These situations may create uncertainty in many aspects of a child's life, including disrupted day-to-day routines, financial hardship or changing care arrangements including foster care, permanent separation from family, or frequent changes in where the child lives.

There may be limited contact between an incarcerated parent and child and potentially a repetition of these disruptions if the parent is in and out of prison. Children may experience the stress response of abandonment, including trust issues or being wary of creating relationships (La Vigne, Davies, & Brazzell 2008).

Children may also have a social stigma or feel shame because of parental incarceration. There may be social backlash from peers or a lack of understanding from adults and service providers in their life (La Vigne, Davies, & Brazzell 2008). There may be additional sources of trauma if children witness the incident that led to the arrest or the arrest itself or are exposed to violence or drug and alcohol use in the community (Youth.gov, n.d.).

A child with an incarcerated parent will most likely feel stress, sadness, or fear and may develop depression or other anxieties. There may be short-term behavioral changes like withdrawal or increased aggression as well as long-term risk for social, emotional, and physical changes.

Research continues to show the importance of strong relationships between children and trusted adults and the role that resilience can play in positive outcomes for children (Joseph & Strain 2010; McNally & Slutsky 2018). Resources created from these findings are used to support children with incarcerated parents. In addition, a continuing pushback against mass incarceration and continued efforts to disrupt the prison pipeline will provide more systemic change.

Deployment

Approximately 1.7 million children in the United States have at least one parent serving in a branch of the military (DMDC 2019). As with any group, not all children in military families have the same experiences, and the impact of their experiences can be very different. In many ways, the stressors are similar to those faced by all young children. However, when a parent is deployed or sent from the place where they are stationed (their home installation) to a specific location for a particular mission, the military service member is separated from their family. Deployment can occur with little notice, making it difficult for children to adjust to the situation. There is also anxiety and fear that the person who is deployed may be in danger since deployments are often for combat operations where it can be difficult to maintain regular contact with them. Changes in the family's living situation during the deployment can upend routines even more.

Even though the military provides a wide support system for the families of deployed service members, the stress on a family is immense. Stress on the parent or guardian who remains can cause trauma for the young children of deployed service members. The more overwhelmed and stressed the parent or guardian feels, the more severe the impact on the child (Cooper & Sogomonyan 2010). Maltreatment severity and risk increase during deployment as well. Neglect rates are two times higher than among families without a family member deployed (James & Countryman 2012), which puts children at risk for additional trauma and traumatic response.

Young children are the most vulnerable to the effects of parental deployment, with those ages 3–5 having the highest reported number of behavioral problems. Military spouses report that children's problem behaviors, anxiety, and stress increase in response to deployment (James & Countryman 2012). These behaviors may include aggression or acting out and anger toward the deployed parent. Other children may withdraw and have intense anxiety and fear related to the person who is away. Children are at greater risk for negative outcomes when a family member has been deployed multiple times or for long stretches, when two parents are deployed, or when the deployed parent is a single parent.

While a substantial number of children experience trauma due to parental deployment, there are many excellent support systems available to military families. Families who feel supported in these ways experience less deployment stress (Cooper & Sogomonyan 2010), and most children in military families do not experience negative outcomes.

Category 4: Violence and Disaster

Violence and disasters are a reality for children no matter their age or where they live. Looking at a few broad examples can help you understand the effects on children and adjust to better meet their needs.

Gun Violence

Gun violence is not a new issue, although it has received more mainstream media coverage attention with the rise in mass shooting events in the United States. Communities have been grappling for years with how to prevent gun violence and support survivors, and the problem is only growing. Early childhood educators need to be a part of the discussion since children are intimately affected by gun violence. An average of 96 people, including 7 children and teens, will die from gun violence *every day* (Everytown, n.d.). In addition, numerous children and teens die by firearm-related suicide each year or are killed each year in unintentional shootings when a child accesses an unsecured gun and kills themselves or someone else (CDC 2015; Everytown, n.d.).

The effects of gun violence are experienced by relatives, friends, community members, and society as a whole, and the loss, fear, safety concerns, and other emotional response can last for a long time.

Natural and Human-Made Disasters

Phenomena such as hurricanes, earthquakes, tornados, floods, and wildfires can cause children to be displaced, their normal routines to be disrupted for long periods of time, and the loss of home or personal items. With entire communities being affected, there can be a loss of community support, creation of economic hardships, and injury and loss of life.

Global pandemics, such as the spread of COVID-19 in 2019–2020, are another form of widespread disruption that affects entire communities and leaves an impact on children. These include economic and social impacts such as loss of work, extended school closures, isolation, and severe illness and loss of life.

The unpredictability of such events—often coming with little warning or chance to prepare—means that children can become extremely fearful of events repeating themselves and want to have as much control over their situation as possible. They may try to keep loved ones or precious belongings close at all times and take extreme preparation measures, like always having emergency kits with them or never playing out of sight of an adult.

Children may regress in behaviors such as having toileting incidents or exhibit changes in sleeping and eating patterns. They may also be clingy and need extra reassurance or have fear and anxiety triggered by reminders of the event. For example, a child who witnessed a wildfire may react when they smell smoke or see a campfire.

Automobile Crashes

Crashes and their aftermath can be extremely frightening, and injury or death is a very real possibility. Traffic collisions are distressingly common; motor vehicle crashes are one of the top three leading causes of unintentional death for children in the United States (Johns Hopkins University, n.d.). Plane and train crashes, while not as frequent, can also be catastrophic and terrifying to those involved and their families since they often happen on a much larger scale and the risk for serious injury or death is high. Children who have been involved in any collision, even a relatively mild car crash, may experience symptoms of PTSD (see page 14).

Personal Injury and Assault or Witnessing Violence

Violence affects children when they are either personally injured or assaulted or witness violence in their home and community. About 51 percent of children report being physically assaulted over their lifetime, and 37 percent report having witnessed violence at some point in their life (Child Trends 2016). This may include experiencing or witnessing maltreatment, sexual assault, or nonfatal assaults or witnessing homicide or intimate partner violence.

Experiencing or witnessing violence has effects that can last well beyond the event itself. Even a single event can undermine children's sense of trust and safety. They may worry about the security of their environment and whether they will be protected at home, in their early childhood program, and in the community. They also may fear for the safety of loved ones or be less willing to trust adults after seeing someone they know and care about being violent. If children feel they are no longer safe, they may switch into survival mode, living with a heightened sense of fear or readiness to protect themselves (NCTSN, n.d. b).

Symptoms can mimic those of PTSD. Children may have behavior changes like being more withdrawn or aggressive. They may try to avoid situations that remind them of the violent event or be more easily startled and have physical complaints like stomachaches and headaches. Some children may also feel responsible for what happened and feel guilty for not taking action or for being safe when others were harmed.

Terrorism

Terrorism is a very particular type of assault rooted in using violence, fear, coercion, or intimidation to achieve a political, economic, religious, or social goal (National Consortium for the Study of Terrorism and Responses to Terrorism [START] 2018). It may be an act of mass violence like a shooting or bombing or a more targeted hate crime designed specifically to hurt or intimidate parts of the population because of prejudice toward their race, cultural background, religion, sexual orientation, or gender identity.

How children are affected by terrorism varies widely depending on the type of event, how much they or their families were personally affected, their understanding of what happened, and what the recovery afterward looks like. For children directly affected by a terrorist attack, the potential for trauma is linked to the other causes we have discussed. They may be personally injured or assaulted or may potentially witness violence in their community. Friends and loved ones may have been hurt or killed, shattering their general sense of safety and security.

Easy access to descriptions, photos, videos, and accounts of terrorist attacks from television, the internet, and other sources means children may view graphic content over and over again. Young children do not have a secure grasp on time and distance, so they may interpret every image as a separate attack or think that faraway events are happening in their neighborhood. This fear is very real and may manifest in trauma symptoms similar to those seen in children who have personally experienced violence.

Post-Traumatic Stress Disorder

PTSD is a specific mental health problem linked closely to all types of traumatic events. Although it was first associated with combat veterans, it may occur in anyone who is exposed to a trauma. People may develop PTSD at any age after experiencing or witnessing a life-threatening event (US Department of Veterans Affairs 2019). It is estimated that 39 percent of preschoolers who have been exposed to trauma will develop PTSD (Fletcher 2003). In fact, since 2013, there is a designated subtype of PTSD known as PTSD for preschool, which describes how the disorder affects children ages 6 and under.

PTSD is characterized by anxiety-related symptoms that develop after exposure to trauma, that worsen over time, last longer than one month, and interfere with day-to-day functioning (US Department of Veterans Affairs 2019). PTSD can last for a brief time or go on for months, years, or the rest of the person's life depending on the severity of the traumatic event and the person's reaction to it.

PTSD symptoms in young children include being irritable or hyperalert, having trouble sleeping and concentrating, being more clingy to trusted and familiar family members, reverting to behaviors they had outgrown like bedwetting and thumb sucking, and re-enacting the trauma or aspects of it through play (Mayo Clinic 2018).

Role of Racism in Trauma and Child Well-Being

Discussion of trauma and young children would be incomplete without specific attention paid to the role of racism in trauma and child health. Racial trauma, or race-based traumatic stress, occurs when people experience or witness racism, whether as microaggressions (see the sidebar), as threats of harm, or as blatant hate crimes and physical assaults (Comas-Díaz, Hall, & Neville 2019; Sue et al. 2007; Williams 2015).

Racism often plays a major role in trauma. Indeed, racism has been identified by the Surgeon General as a cause of trauma (Carter 2006). Children of different races are exposed to trauma at different rates. A 2018 study (Wamser-Nanney et al.) found that Black children are more likely to be exposed to multiple types of trauma, experience more community violence, and be placed in protective custody more frequently than White children. Black and Latino children are at higher risk for child maltreatment, chiefly witnessing domestic violence (Roberts et al. 2011).

ACEs, too, vary by race and ethnicity. In the United States, 61 percent of Black children and 51 percent of Latino children have experienced at least one ACE, compared with 40 percent of White children and 23 percent of Asian children (Sacks & Murphey 2018). ACEs do not exist in isolation; they often occur because of systems in place that perpetuate cycles of disadvantage, oppression, and violence.

Statistics on incidence and reaction to trauma are just part of the picture. Racism can affect children on many levels. These include structural disadvantages through ongoing neighborhood and school segregation, which unevenly distribute resources (Reskin 2012). Discrimination puts Black, Latino, and Native Americans at a greater risk of either being poor or living in poor neighborhoods because of factors related to racist practices in housing and the job market. Living in poor neighborhoods likewise opens families up to ACEs linked to poverty (Child Trends 2019).

Racism also exists on a personally mediated level where a child's abilities and motives are assumed because of their race (Trent, Dooley, & Dougé 2019). In early childhood education this can be seen explicitly through studies such as the one conducted at Yale Child Study Center that showed that preschool teachers already had an implicit bias against young Black boys that was evident in their interpretation of challenging behaviors and the expectations they had for the children (Gilliam et al. 2016).

How racism intersects with trauma is not limited to firsthand experiences. Historical trauma is a form of trauma that affects an entire community across multiple generations. It is often linked with racial and ethnic population groups that have experienced major intergenerational losses and assaults on their culture and well-being. This includes the legacy of enslaved Africans who were forcefully relocated to the United States, Native Americans who were displaced and murdered, and Jews who were exterminated or survived the concentration camps of the Holocaust (ACF, n.d. b; NCTSN 2017).

Historical trauma has a psychological and emotional response that is felt by descendants, families, and communities. In addition, researchers have found that descendants of those who experienced group genocide and experiences like slavery have inherited biological changes in response to trauma, such as heightened stress responses (NCTSN 2017). This then changes the way the body interprets and responds to stressful incidents. Historical trauma can negatively affect the physical, psychological, and social health of individuals and entire communities that share a past history of racial hatred and genocide (Resler 2019).

In addition, groups continue to be the target of persecution and hate in a way that is directly linked to the historical targeting. Ongoing discrimination in the labor market, policing, and education, for example, motivates many parents to prepare their children for the risk of experiencing discrimination. The day-to-day stress of living with discrimination can have significant physical effects (Chatterjee & Davis 2017).

Families affected by historical trauma often have personal, cultural, and community strengths that enable them to be resilient. However, historical trauma is an important perspective when considering how children, families, and educators are affected by traumatic incidents, and it is critical that early childhood educators understand what they can do to provide a welcoming, fair environment for all children and families (see Chapter 6).

Microaggressions

Microaggressions are "daily verbal, visual, behavioral, or environmental indignities" toward people of color that "communicate hostile, derogatory, or negative racial slights and insults" (Sue et al. 2007, 271). A microaggression might involve name calling, such as "colored," "Oriental," or "you people." It conveys rudeness or insensitivity, for example, telling a job applicant of color, " I believe the most qualified person should get the job, regardless of race" or a White teacher ignoring children of color when listening to children at group time. Microaggressions exclude or nullify the feelings and experiences of a person of color, such as occurs when complimenting a person on their English or saying, "When I look at you, I don't see color."

In early childhood education, microaggression is often manifest in a learning environment where books, materials, room decorations, and photos reflect only the dominant culture and where children of color, especially Black boys, are unfairly targeted as disruptive or the perpetuators of anything that goes wrong (Friedman & Mwenelupembe 2020).

What makes this type of racial trauma particularly insidious is that microaggressions often operate below the surface. They may be inflicted unintentionally by those unaware that their words are causing offense and pain. But as early childhood teacher Bret Turner (2019) notes, "At their core, [microaggressions] are coded messages of disapproval that are based in identity: comments and actions that echo larger, structural bigotry, telling marginalized people they don't belong, that they are less than. Children start internalizing these messages while they are still developing their identities."

The Influence of Other Factors on Children's Experiences of Trauma

Other factors that intersect with trauma in addition to race and poverty include culture, disability, and gender.

Culture

Culture includes the set of behaviors, values, and traditions shared by a group of people. It is a lens that frames children's understanding of events and shapes their processing of trauma as well as their reactions to it (Caspi et al. 2013). Culture also influences children's ability to show resilience in the face of trauma.

People of different cultures may define trauma differently and use different expressions to describe their experiences (NCTSN 2013). Each child has unique experiences and cultural expectations, and educators need to understand children's ways of expressing their experiences. Families in some cultures may avoid disclosure of abuse and other ACEs because it would prove embarrassing if known (Collin-Vezina, Daigneault, & Hébert 2013) and would make the families negatively stand out within their communities. Children in these cultures may learn to internalize their feelings. In some cultures or communities, people are less likely to actively pursue treatment related to trauma recovery (NCTSN 2010). Children in these cultures may be reluctant to share their feelings and may even be shamed by family members if they react to trauma. Still other children are from cultures that work to upend ACEs.

Culture influences how each child reacts to the same trauma. Consider this pre-K classroom:

> Four-year-old Jae-Joong, who is Korean American, believes that to be respectful to his teacher, he should not express his feelings and fears concerning the recent shooting in his neighborhood that killed a 14-year-old Latino boy. Instead, he withdraws into himself and shows little interest in classroom activities.
>
> In contrast, his 4-year-old classmate Darius, whose family is from Trinidad and Tobago and who lives in Jae-Joong's neighborhood, has always been encouraged to express his feelings. With wide eyes and expressive hand gestures, Darius relates everything he knows about the shooting to his teacher. During the next several days, he repeats his tale and re-enacts the incident, focusing on little else.

While Darius's teachers may readily understand that Darius is dealing with the aftereffects of trauma, they may not be as insightful about Jae-Joong. It may take careful observation and skill to see that he too is in need of immediate attention. Both boys are dealing with trauma in the only way they know how. Both need assistance from their teachers to come to terms with what they have experienced. Until then, neither child will be able to focus on learning.

Learn to know the children's families well and appreciate their cultural values and norms. This knowledge will help you to better understand how children who have gone through trauma may internalize the experience.

Disability

Children with some disabilities are more predisposed to experiencing ACEs than are their peers without these disabilities. For example, children with intellectual and developmental disabilities (IDD) are at greater risk for experiencing ACEs, such as abuse and neglect, than are children without these impairments (NCTSN 2016). Because these children are at high risk for trauma, "any behavior . . . could be an expression of trauma versus something that just comes along with their disability" (NCTSN 2016, 1).

There is great overlap in behaviors expressed by children who have experienced trauma and children with diagnosed disabilities or conditions such as autism, attention-deficit/hyperactivity disorder (ADHD), emotional disturbance, oppositional defiance disorder, sensory integration disorder, IDD, depression, and anxiety (Nicholson, Perez, & Kurtz 2019). This causes some children who have experienced trauma to receive such misdiagnoses as ADHD, and vice versa (Miller 2014). Children who have been neglected or abused often have difficulty forming relationships with teachers and other adults; have chronic dysregulation (that is, difficulty regulating their emotions and behavior); think negatively; are hypervigilant; and are inattentive, hyperactive, and impulsive (Miller, n.d.). These symptoms are also typically associated with ADHD. So while some children who have experienced trauma may actually have ADHD, many others have received incorrect diagnoses. To further exacerbate this, a child who receives an incorrect diagnosis of ADHD and the typical ADHD treatment of behavioral therapy and stimulant medication will not experience symptom relief since the root cause is trauma.

By addressing the role trauma has played in the child's behaviors, the child's evaluation team can determine whether or not trauma is at the root of the problem, thus preventing a misdiagnosis (Crecco, n.d.). At the same time, staff can make sure that a child with a history of trauma who also has an identifiable disability such as ADHD or IDD has a treatment plan that outlines both the socioemotional supports the child needs to address the roots of trauma and the supports needed to address the disability.

Gender

Gender also plays a role in how young children experience and are affected by trauma. Girls are more prone to experiencing ACEs in all categories than boys; sexual trauma and physical punishment are especially more common in girls than boys (Epstein & Gonzalez, n.d.). Boys are more likely to experience nonsexual assaults, traffic collisions, and injuries and to witness violence than are girls (Ziegler 2011). And while transgendered youth are not identified in studies at ages 3–6, young people who identify as transgender were found to be 28 percent more likely to experience physical violence than those who identify as cisgender (Treleaven 2018).

Researchers have also found gender differences in children's reactions and resilience from trauma. Girls are more prone to internalizing their reactions through depression and anxiety following trauma, while boys show more anger and dissociation (Foster, Kuperminc, & Price 2004). Furthermore, boys have a stronger response to firsthand trauma than to secondhand trauma. Girls' responses are equally strong when exposed to either firsthand or secondhand trauma (NCCD Center for Girls and Young Women, n.d.).

Responses to Trauma Are Individual

The experiences and events outlined in this chapter have the capacity to cause trauma response in children, but not all children who have these experiences will exhibit a traumatic response. Children respond to adverse events in different ways. Some will show signs of traumatic response as soon as the events occur, while others may act normally for a while and then show symptoms of traumatic response weeks or even months later.

The intensity and lasting power of the traumatic response in children depends on several factors. The nature of the traumatic event, for example, has great bearing on how deeply the effects of the trauma are felt. Being in a traffic collision where no one is seriously injured may not lead to behavioral symptoms. Indeed, most children have the resilience to bounce back from one traumatic incident and return to their normal level of functioning (Presidential Task Force on Posttraumatic Stress Disorder and Trauma in Children and Adolescents 2008). However, if the one-time trauma is horrific, such as a child witnessing a loved one being killed, it is more likely to leave deep scarring and serious ongoing symptoms.

Other factors such as the child's temperament, their age when the trauma began or was experienced, how long the trauma persisted, whether the trauma was experienced firsthand or secondhand, the presence of other risk factors (for example, poverty, a parent's mental health, community violence), and the child's support system and level of resilience all influence how a child responds.

It is critical to not simply look at a list of potential triggers to decide whether a child has or has not experienced trauma. Take into consideration the severity of the problem; individual factors such as the child's age, development, and disabilities or developmental delays; the child's perception and emotional reaction, and whether family members recognize the source of the child's distress and are actively seeking ways to alleviate the dysfunction.

It is also important to remember that although you play a vital role in supporting children and families and in providing nurturing environments that help children heal and thrive, you are *not* a specialist in diagnosing conditions or treating children who have been severely affected by trauma. Moreover, while the signs discussed in this chapter are often a response to trauma, a child may exhibit these behaviors because of another cause. Working closely with families, other primary support systems, and specialists is critical to ensure that children receive the care they need.

A Path Forward

Creating a safe environment with consistent routines and establishing trusting, strong relationships gives educators numerous tools they can employ with the children they work with. Future chapters will talk in depth about these ideas and how they can be applied in your program. To lay the groundwork for those strategies, in the next chapter, we look at the ways trauma can affect children's development. Combined with the information you have learned about types of trauma, this will help you to see how the physical, mental, and social consequences of trauma overlap.

Three

How Trauma Affects Young Children's Brains and Their Ability to Learn

The child behaviors that challenge and puzzle educators are often the only tools a child has for processing adverse experiences. The behaviors also indicate what is happening in the brain. While a discussion of such a complex topic as brain development is beyond the scope of this book, understanding basic ways trauma can affect a child's brain can help you as you partner with families and others to find the most effective ways to support children's healthy growth and development.

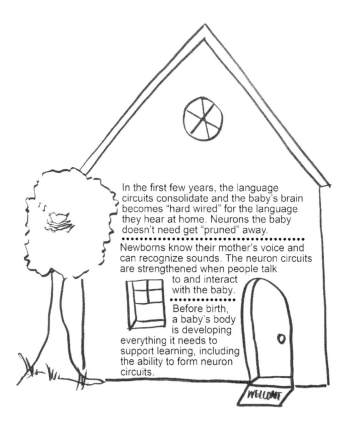

In the first few years, the language circuits consolidate and the baby's brain becomes "hard wired" for the language they hear at home. Neurons the baby doesn't need get "pruned" away.

Newborns know their mother's voice and can recognize sounds. The neuron circuits are strengthened when people talk to and interact with the baby.

Before birth, a baby's body is developing everything it needs to support learning, including the ability to form neuron circuits.

Figure 1. Just like a house, brain functions are built level by level.

Brain Circuits and Connections

Brain development is not a straightforward march along a set pathway. It is an interactive process in which genes provide a blueprint and experiences customize the brain to function in its particular environment (Center on the Developing Child, n.d. b; Sorrels 2015).

Neuronal connections, or circuits, build over time from simple connections into more complex interactions. In the first few years of life, "more than 1 million new neuronal connections form every second" (Center on the Developing Child, n.d. b). There is a reason the process of brain development is known as "brain architecture" (Center on the Developing Child, n.d. b): the process is similar to building a house, and it starts with a strong foundation (see Fig. 1).

Neuronal connections are either strengthened by repeated use or discarded if they are not needed. The process of discarding underused neuronal connections is called *pruning* and represents the brain fine-tuning the connections to be as adaptable as possible in response to environmental stimuli. A flexible brain can better take in and process information and adjust to thrive within the environment (Rotshtein & Mitchell 2018).

Experience and Brain Connections

A child's early experiences—such as sensory input and the ability to explore and interact with the world—play a huge role in determining which connections are strengthened and which are pruned (Rotshtein & Mitchell 2018). For example, if a child is not exposed to rich and varied vocabulary or allowed to actively explore the environment, some of the neuronal networks needed for cognitive or academic learning may be pruned away (Nicholson, Perez, & Kurtz 2019). In the first few years of life, the brain is creating the foundation for all future learning, including social, emotional, and communication skills, by building strong neuronal connections that allow the brain to take in and use information and build on existing patterns and knowledge. Having a healthy, supportive environment is critical to this process since it allows the brain to physically develop.

For example, one way neuronal connections are strengthened is through serve-and-return interactions between a child and another individual (see Fig. 2). These occur when an infant or young child babbles, gestures, cries, or otherwise engages with people and objects around them and an older child or adult responds through eye contact, words, physical contact like hugs, or other responsive actions. At the brain level, this back-and-forth strengthens the neuronal connections; at the behavioral level, the interaction builds crucial communication and social skills (Center on the Developing Child, n.d. d). Without this environmental feedback, young children may not develop these skills, because the neuronal connections aren't strengthened and may eventually be pruned if they are underused. This means there is not as robust a foundation for developing future skills.

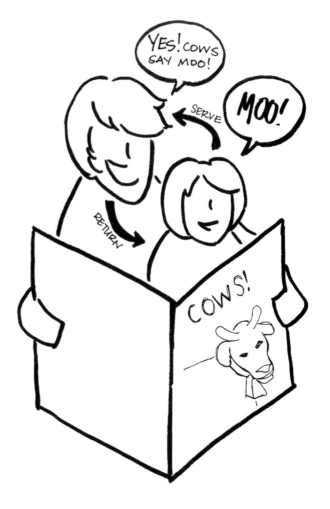

Figure 2. A serve-and-return interaction.

Responding to Stress

Adults not only help shape a child's brain development through the interactions and experiences they provide, they also play an important role in helping children learn how to react and deal with difficult situations and develop a healthy stress response. Normal stress responses are brief, allowing the body to return to its natural state or baseline. For example, a child who is momentarily startled or frightened by someone saying "boo" may experience an increase in heart rate and breathe more rapidly. For most children that will last for only a few moments, and then they will return to their usual state of regulation.

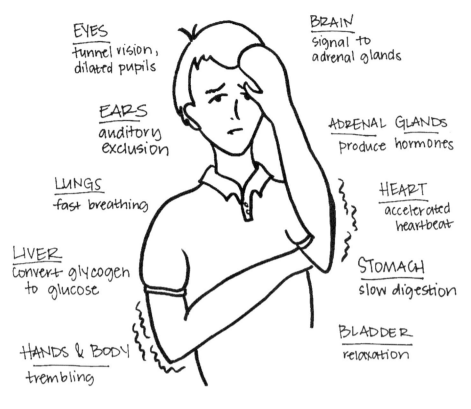

EYES
tunnel vision, dilated pupils

EARS
auditory exclusion

LUNGS
fast breathing

LIVER
convert glycogen to glucose

HANDS & BODY
trembling

BRAIN
signal to adrenal glands

ADRENAL GLANDS
produce hormones

HEART
accelerated heartbeat

STOMACH
slow digestion

BLADDER
relaxation

Figure 3. The body's reactions to stress.

States of prolonged stress in children may occur after more severe traumas, like threat of physical or emotional harm, a severe injury, or the death of a loved one. At these times, a child's body reacts by increasing the heart rate and blood pressure and releasing stress hormones (see Fig. 3). The longer the impact of the trauma, the longer these reactions last (Center on the Developing Child, n.d. e).

Learning to cope with these physiological changes in a healthy way is critical for children so they gain the skills they need to respond to stress or discomfort and can adapt and remain in control of their reaction. Children develop these skills by having caring adults model healthy reactions to stress and provide safe spaces where children can practice these skills. For example, you might encourage a child who is feeling angry to pound playdough, do some jumping jacks, or punch a pillow. Help the child find what works for them. When you teach a child how to deal with the stress in healthy ways, and the underlying conflict is resolved, the child's body can adapt and return to its baseline state. Strategies for helping children regulate their emotional state are detailed in Chapter 4.

If trauma is complex or repeated, like physical or emotional abuse, and if supportive adults aren't consistently present to help the child due to factors like neglect, family separation, mental illness, or substance use, a child's body can experience a sustained stress response, known as *toxic stress*. In response, the brain sends signals for the body to take action in one of these ways: fight, flight, or freeze (Texas Children's Hospital 2019). Instead of focusing on building healthy, strong neuronal connections— including those relating to the development of higher-order thinking skills—the brain puts its energy into a protective response (Center on the Developing Child, n.d. b). Figure 4, on the next page, illustrates the difference between the types of stress response.

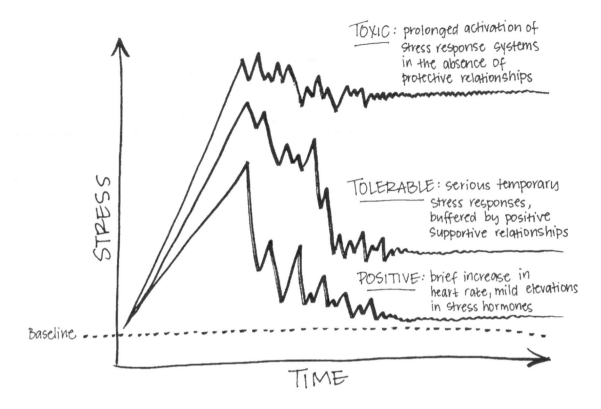

Figure 4. Types of stress response.

The Impact of Trauma on Development and Learning

If toxic stress is not alleviated or a child does not receive treatment, the child is at risk for developmental and learning deficits now and for problems in learning, behavior, physical health, and mental well-being into their adulthood (Center on the Developing Child, n.d. e).

Early trauma may lead to documented social and emotional difficulties, such as feelings of hopelessness and helplessness, low self-concept, poor social skills, anxiety, depression, and pessimism. Physically, trauma may interfere with present growth and development and predispose children to lifelong health challenges.

"Effects of Trauma on Development," on page 23, lists possible developmental and learning consequences of toxic stress on young children's cognitive, language, social and emotional, and physical abilities.

What Toxic Stress Looks Like in Early Childhood Programs

In an effort to escape danger and return to a pretrauma safe state, the brain triggers a fight (confront the threat), flight (run away), or freeze (shut down) response. The children in your program may display symptoms of trauma that reflect any of these responses. Though these symptoms may look like intentional misbehavior, they are children's biological responses to the traumas they have endured.

The following behaviors are common signs of toxic stress in very young children (Children's Bureau 2016; Government of Western Australia, n.d.; NCTSN 2008b; Nemeth & Brillante 2011; Sorrels 2015). Keep in mind that children may exhibit some of these signs, to a lesser degree or over a shorter time period, for reasons other than trauma.

Effects of Trauma on Development

Area of Development or Learning	Consequences of Trauma
Cognition and academic learning	Can prevent a child from focusing attention, sequencing thought, and solving problems. Diminishes confidence and can affect ability to enter and sustain dramatic play scenarios.
Language and communication	Affects development of vocabulary, processing of language, communication, self-talk, and conversational skills.
Social and emotional development	Interferes with development of social skills, including respecting boundaries, not being able to take others' perspective into account, and resolving conflict. Can also disrupt the sense of trust and security or cause a child to be in a constant state of fear or anxiety.
Physical development	Can lead to delays or stunted gross motor and fine motor development and negatively affect body awareness and muscle tone.

Fight Behaviors

> **Self-harm,** such as biting oneself, pulling one's hair, banging one's head: Three-year-old Colton gets easily upset when there are changes in the program's routine. When there is a substitute teacher, he goes to a corner of the room and starts hitting his head against the wall. He refuses to be soothed or calmed by the new teacher.

> **Inconsolable or rage-filled crying and tantrums:** When 4-year-old Antonio's friend John tells him he doesn't want to play with him, Antonio starts crying and yelling at John that he hates him. Antonio's crying intensifies and lasts for the rest of free play, despite other friends and his teachers trying to redirect his attention.

> **Inability to be soothed or calmed down:** When the building Merry is working on in the block corner falls, she collapses into a heap on the floor and sobs. Her teacher, Ms. Cunningham, hugs Merry, who continues sobbing in her arms for a long time.

> **Hitting, biting, and other aggressive behavior:** When 3-year-old Shana's friend Paul asks to use the easel she is painting at, Shana hits Paul and shoves the easel toward him, knocking him over.

> **Verbal abuse of others:** When Lamar joins 6-year-old David outside during kindergarten recess, David turns to him and yells, "Get off.

I'm playing here, Stupidface. I didn't tell you you could be here!" Every time Lamar tries to play in the area, David continues yelling at him and calling him names. When a teacher intervenes, David says, "He's dumb and ugly. He can't play with me." This behavior continues for several recess times.

> **Rude or defiant behavior:** When 4-year-old Nathan's teacher announces that it's time to clean up while he's still building with blocks, Nathan announces, "You can't tell me what to do. You're not the boss of me." He continues to build with the blocks despite several verbal warnings. When the teacher comes over to intervene, Nathan kicks the blocks toward her and runs out of the room.

> **Need for more control:** Four-year-old Julian is operating the mouse while sitting at the computer working on a drawing program with Seseko. Seseko asks Julian to use a coloring option to change the background. Without looking at Seseko, Julian grits his teeth and announces, "No. I'm in charge. I have the mouse, so I can do what I want." When Seseko protests, Julian shoves her aside and announces, "I'm the boss. I can do whatever I want. You need to listen to me."

> **Inappropriate sexual behavior or play:** While playing in the dramatic play center, 4-year-old Ramon picks up a girl doll and a boy doll. He then puts the boy doll on top of the girl doll and moves the boy doll up and down over the girl doll while laughing.

Flight Behaviors

> **Separation anxiety** from family or program at arrival or departure: Four-year-old Eduardo cries every morning when his mom drops him off at school, even after being in pre-K for several months.

> **Regression in skills** previously mastered: When 3-year-old James arrives at his program, he turns to his teacher for help taking off his jacket and gloves, activities he was able to do until last week.

> **Loss of bladder control (enuresis):** Five-year-old Samanda has started wetting her pants for the first time all year.

> **Physical complaints** that seem unrelated to illness or accident: Five-year-old Keisha tells her teacher that she has a stomachache nearly every day before going home.

> **Significant changes in eating patterns:** Four-year-old Dougie sits at the table with everyone in his family child care program for lunch, but for the last few days he has refused to take a bite of any of the foods being served.

> **Significant changes in sleep patterns:** Three-year-old Liam lies down on his mat at rest time, gets up to get a toy, lies down again, says he forgot to brush his teeth even though he already brushed them, lies down again, gets up to drink water, and then goes and sits at a table.

> **Worries about their own or another's safety:** Five-year-old Brandy tells her teacher about the drawing she just completed: "The mommy is staying home with her little girl. If she leaves the house, something bad will happen to the little girl."

> **Heightened vigilance** and inaccurate perception of danger: Six-year-old Cecily hears a loud car exhaust sound and runs to take cover.

> **Increased fearfulness:** Three-year-old Montana wakes up from her nap crying and tells her teacher, "There was a monster in the room who was going to eat me."

> **Mood swings and personality changes:** While marching with instruments outside, 4-year-old Marcus happily shakes maracas to the music. Then, without instigation, Marcus throws the maracas on the ground and starts complaining the activity is dumb.

> **Repetitive play that re-creates traumatic events** and is unproductive, not providing relief or further upsetting the child: Following a recent tornado, 4-year-old Giacinta builds a barn out of blocks. Then with a whooshing sound she yells, "Take cover!" and knocks her construction down with one swoop of her arm. She repeats this play over and over throughout the morning, bringing in small dolls and having the "mommy" doll pick up the "baby" doll and run away.

> **Expressing worry that the trauma will recur:** During morning meeting on the anniversary of the date his mother was severely injured in a car crash, 5-year-old Yahir announces that no one should get in a car today.

> **Negative thinking in worst-case scenarios:** When his teacher suggests that 6-year-old Dev join his friends in play on the outdoor equipment, Dev mutters, "They don't want to play with me. They hate me. No one likes me."

> **Frequent talk about death and dying:** While putting on a puppet show with two friends, 3-year-old Brooklyn suggests that the frog puppets go to the funeral for their babysitter who died. When one of the children suggests the puppets go to the movies instead, Brooklyn insists that funerals are more important. No matter what play scenarios the other children begin, Brooklyn always turns it toward a funeral.

Freeze Behaviors

> **Muteness, refusal to talk:** Every day at morning meeting, Ms. Sanchez goes around the circle and has everyone tell the group one thing they would like to do today. Whenever it's Marta's turn, she says nothing. Ms. Sanchez encourages Marta to say something, but Marta sits silently, staring at her teacher with her mouth clenched.

> **Limited eye contact:** When her favorite school bus driver greets her, 6-year-old Keine bows her head and refuses to look him in the eye and give him a big smile as she typically does.

> **Withdrawal from activities:** Five-year-old Emma sits quietly at the morning meeting with her hands in her lap. She stares blankly out the window and doesn't move her head or eyes when the teacher asks for a volunteer to feed the classroom fish.

> **Difficulty forming friendships:** Before going on a nature walk, Mr. Lopez asks the class to find a partner to hold hands with on the walk. As the children pair up, 5-year-old Carmelo just stands there, not making eye contact with anyone. Seeing Carmelo standing alone, Mr. Lopez asks Emmit to be Carmelo's partner. Emmit goes over to Carmelo and extends his hand. Carmelo just stands there as Emmit grabs his hand.

> **Ignoring directions, not listening, or refusing to participate in activities:** While baking bread in a small group, the teacher asks 4-year-old Emilia to proof the yeast by putting it in the bowl of water and sugar on the counter. Emilia takes the package and empties it on the counter. The teacher corrects her, telling her that she needs to clean up the poured yeast and then put another packet in the water. Emilia looks at her teacher and walks away from the cooking center.

> **Quick to give up or unwilling to try new things:** Five-year-old Curtis is working on a puzzle at a table. He puts one piece in and picks up a second piece. He tries it in one spot, but it doesn't fit. He pushes the puzzle away and retreats to the library area.

> **Over- or under-reacting to physical touch:** When it's time to go outside to play, a parent volunteer sees 6-year-old Zara struggling to put on her jacket. The parent walks over to Zara, reaches toward her, and says, "Here, Zara, I can help you." Zara instantly recoils and moves out of reach.

> **Overreacting to sounds or textures:** While having family-style lunch, Ms. Cella passes the food around the table. She encourages 4-year-old Trinity to try some ramen. Trinity reluctantly puts a forkful in her mouth and immediately spits it out: "It's too wiggly and slimy. It feels yucky in my mouth."

> **Overly dependent on others:** Four-year-old Carola often insists that her teacher help her with tasks that she could easily do herself. When a parent volunteer attempts to get out her cot for rest time, Carola snaps at her, "I want Ms. Knight to help me. She knows how to do it."

> **Lack of self-confidence:** While playing outdoors, Mr. Louis asks 6-year-old Connor to catch the ball with him. Connor softly replies, "I can't do it. I can't do anything."

Some children exposed to toxic stress will exhibit just one or two signs while others will show multiple symptoms. It is important to remember that you are not responsible for confirming whether a child is dealing with toxic stress or providing any sort of diagnosis. These signs and examples can help you recognize that sometimes behaviors are a result of trauma, not a child's intentional misbehavior or temporary circumstances. If you see these types of challenging behaviors, you can begin to help the child regulate their emotions using the strategies presented in Chapters 4–7.

A Path Forward

Understanding how children's brain development and trauma are related and being able to identify what sort of physical, emotional, and social cues a child may exhibit if they are having a traumatic response will focus your efforts on helping the child in the moment. In addition, knowing some basics about brain development and the influence of early experiences will give you the tools to help others, such as family members, administrators, or lawmakers, understand the critical importance of TIC. The next few chapters will give you specific strategies to incorporate into your program to support children and families.

CHAPTER Four

Guiding Principles for Teaching Children with Trauma

Although many educators feel that young children will outgrow the effects of trauma, this is a mistaken belief. Young children are both the most vulnerable of populations and the most deeply influenced by trauma (Nicholson, Perez, & Kurtz 2019).

> Three-year-old Liam has never had trouble falling asleep during rest time. Even after wildfires forced his family to flee their home six weeks ago, Liam has slept well, hugging his stuffed penguin, Pablo, closely to his tummy. Lately though, Liam has become anxious as rest time approaches. His educator, Ms. Sherrow, shares her concern with Liam's mom: "It's almost like he is scared to fall asleep." Ms. Sherrow is observing that signs of trauma may lay dormant and suddenly appear well after the trauma itself has ended.

. . . .

> Five-year-old Emma has never missed a day of school. At the home visit before kindergarten started, Emma's grandmother, with whom she lives, shared with her teacher, Ms. Garcia, that Emma had been sexually abused by a family member when she was 2 and 3 years old. Ms. Garcia is surprised that despite the severe trauma in her life, Emma never acts out in the classroom. In fact, she seems to be in her own world, often staring into space. Emma keeps to herself and never bothers anyone. What Ms. Garcia has not yet realized is that Emma's withdrawal and daydreaming are very much signs of trauma, too.

Experiences like Liam's and Emma's are not unique. Children are not immune to aftereffects from natural disasters, abuse, and other adverse experiences. As you've read in the previous chapters, trauma negatively affects children's developing brains and bodies and has the potential to cause lifelong damage.

However, over the last 20 years or so, much has been learned about trauma and how a healing-centered approach can help children recover from these negative experiences. Indeed, coupling your expertise with the support of colleagues, specialists, families, and community leaders has the potential to ensure that children are not doomed by their past.

In this chapter we offer foundational information on basic principles that can be used to inform and guide your interactions with children. Chapters 5, 6, and 7 will discuss how to use these approaches in your day-to-day teaching practice. The following principles offer overarching guidance on teaching children exposed to trauma.

Principle 1: Recognize that All Children Will Benefit from a Trauma-Informed Approach

TIC focuses on social and emotional supports to help children learn to self-calm, regulate their emotions, and focus on learning. It is rooted in relationships and trust and emphasizes safety, predictability, and consistency. These are important social and emotional supports for *every* young child, so using a trauma-informed approach serves everyone in your program. By supporting the development of skills such as executive function, making friends, problem solving, and empathy, you are readying every child you teach for learning and school success.

As noted in Chapter 1, you may not be certain whether a child has been affected by trauma or not. Not all instances of trauma are readily identifiable. Some children with ACEs may be known to you because the child welfare system is involved in their lives. However, some children with ACEs may never be known to you. While it is possible with parental permission to screen all children in your program for trauma and then link the results to service delivery systems such as a multitiered system of support (MTSS), doing so is a debatable approach. As of 2016, only one in eight schools at every level in the United States was making use of universal screening (Eklund & Rossen 2016).

In this book, we do not recommend the use of universal screening by schools or programs. For one thing, screening can lead to embarrassment or shame. Being known as a child who receives special treatment sets one apart from one's peers. Since one of the primary goals of recovery is to normalize life for a child exposed to trauma, no child should feel less than normal because of what they have experienced in life. "The best approach is to make sure we provide trauma-sensitive learning environments for *all* children" (Cole et al. 2013, 9).

Even when educators are aware of specific children having experienced trauma, they cannot assume that they know the extent of the children's traumas or the underlying causes. Very often there is more to the story that hasn't been uncovered. As the Council for Professional Recognition (2019) cautions early childhood educators, "You don't need to know exactly what caused the trauma to be able to help. Instead of focusing on the specifics of a stressful situation, concentrate on the support you can give. Stick with what you see—the hurt, anger, and worry—instead of getting every detail of a child's story" (6).

Providing the same social and emotional supports to all children in your classroom or family child care program will help ensure that no child who has experienced trauma will slip through the cracks. And every child will be enriched by your sensitive asset-building teaching.

Principle 2: Use a Strengths-Based Approach to Teaching

A natural impulse for many educators is to assess what a child's problems are and then try to fix them. You may even wonder whether children so traumatized by their experiences can ever become healthy. Yet when working with children who have been frightened and disoriented by immigration experiences, beaten down by abuse, or depressed by loss, focusing on what's wrong both makes the problems worse and tends to leave children disengaged (Lewis 2015). Instead of focusing on what a child is lacking, build on what the child knows and can do. Strengths-based teaching has educators help children assess what they do well and then use these strengths and talents to build and bridge knowledge. You do this by focusing on the following (Zacarian, Alvarez-Ortiz, & Haynes 2017b):

> Identifying children's existing strengths

> Honoring, valuing, and acknowledging these strengths

> Helping students become aware of their strengths

> Building instructional programming that boosts social ties and networks by drawing from children's strengths

Drawing on children's strengths and capacities builds resilience and helps them develop the skills, competencies, and confidence they need to become active learners and critical thinkers. It also leads to improved educational outcomes, more success, increased engagement, and even greater happiness (Biswas-Diener, Kashdan, & Gurpal 2011; Ginwright 2018; SAMHSA 2014b; Zacarian, Alvarez-Ortiz, & Haynes 2017b). This doesn't mean that you deny the existence of barriers and challenges to the children's learning, but that you use your energy and attention to intentionally focus on children's assets.

You'll find that it doesn't take great effort to identify strengths in young children, even when trauma has left them with great challenges. So much growth and development take place during the preschool and kindergarten years that there is always some new strength and capacity that emerges: "You sang 'Itsy, Bitsy Spider' all by yourself, Anyah! Maybe you and Keily would like to sing the song to all of us at our afternoon meeting."

Strengths-based teaching is especially well suited to children who have had trauma in their lives (Zacarian, Alvarez-Ortiz, & Haynes 2017a). It allows educators to focus on the whole child rather than the trauma or the child's behavior. This means looking at the child's personality, relationships, family and community values and beliefs, interests and dislikes, protective factors, support systems, and other capacities (Nicholson, Perez, & Kurtz 2019).

Proponents of a strengths-based approach envision children's assets as being like individual tiles in a mosaic. Each strength may not stand out individually, but all the tiles taken together become a unified piece of art (Zacarian, Alvarez-Ortiz, & Haynes 2017a). As an educator, your mission is to take all a child's individual tiles—or assets—and use them as a foundation for helping that child learn and succeed.

Principle 3: Recognize, Appreciate, and Address Differing Influences on Children's Experiences with Trauma

Chapter 2 discussed some of the ways factors such as race, culture, language, socioeconomic status, disability, and gender influence the experience of trauma for children and how bias and discrimination in response to such aspects of children's identities can be a source of trauma (Carter 2006; Hughes & Tucker 2018; Stevens 2015). A key part of individualizing your approach and making use of trauma-sensitive guidelines is to view children's experiences through these lenses. While none of these influences predetermine a child's response, they are an important part of the picture when determining how to best reach and teach individual children.

Here are some fundamental actions you can take as you seek to better understand the influences on individual children's experience of trauma:

> Get to know every family and child well. Understanding another person can strip away stereotypes and replace them with respect, understanding, and appreciation of differences as well as similarities. Do not assume that people who share a cultural or other identity have the same experiences or follow the same traditions. Knowing the specific country a family has emigrated from, for instance, is helpful in better understanding that family. Even more helpful is learning to know their individual experiences and practices.

> Know yourself. Examine your own biases for preconceived notions and ways in which your own background and experiences might influence how you interact with children and families. Reflect on the language (both spoken and body language) you use to make sure that you are not inflicting microaggressions (see Chapter 2). Videorecord yourself during children's play and group times to study your responses to children to determine any biases you may be acting on.

> Support children's identities through books, music, toys and other materials, language, and cooking experiences that reflect the children, families, and their communities. Have dress-up clothes and props for dramatic play that are familiar to children, including open-ended pieces that can be used in multiple ways and items that are representative of their communities. Encourage children to have pride in who they are and to appreciate others for who they are.

> Read aloud, discuss, and have children act out in skits and with puppets storybooks that deal with trauma through specific lenses such as race, culture, or gender. For example, *Ouch! Moments: When Words Are Used in Hurtful Ways* (by Michael Genhart) addresses racial microaggressions.

> Work to forge a bond with each child, bearing in mind how factors like differences in home language, culture, and race may affect your interactions and the child's responses. Designate one-on-one time every day.

> Offer play experiences that children can participate in regardless of language. Art, sand and water play, and music are open-ended experiences where all children can express themselves.

> Connect with community groups that serve migrant and refugee families for ongoing support, ideas, and knowledge of how to better serve families in their home languages.

> For children with disabilities or developmental delays, who often need predictability to be successful, avoid changes to the daily routine and environment as much as possible to alleviate the stress that children often experience following trauma (CDC 2019). Offer soothing sensory techniques such as drawing, deep breathing, mindfulness, yoga, or exercising to manage emotions. As described in Principles 5 and 6, focus on building children's self-regulation skills, not just working to reduce challenging behaviors (Rossen 2018).

> While children display a variety of reactions to trauma, keep in mind that that there are gender differences in children's reactions to trauma and their resilience. In general, girls experience depression and anxiety following trauma, while boys show more anger and act aggressively (Epstein & Gonzalez, n.d; Foster, Kuperminc, & Price 2004). Mindfulness is an important strategy for helping children regardless of gender develop needed self-regulation. See Chapter 6 for more on mindfulness.

> Perhaps most important, be an advocate for all children and families, particularly those whose experience of trauma may be affected by the factors discussed here. Chapter 8 suggests several ways you can do this.

Principle 4: Embrace Resilience as a Goal for Every Child

As an educator, you want many things for children: to master the goals in the curriculum; to develop a love of learning and a sense of curiosity; to be creative; to think critically; to appreciate the arts; to be kind and empathic; to make responsible decisions and solve problems; to feel capable, competent, and confident; to be able to reach their full potential; and to feel optimistic about themselves, others, and the world they live in. Touching on all these goals is a desire for children to be resilient—to be able to overcome whatever adversities they have been exposed to so they can learn and reach their full potential. It's important that even children who have not been exposed to trauma be resilient so that they are prepared for whatever challenges life throws their way.

Culture is among the factors that influence children's resilience, and it has a strong influence on both a child's reaction to trauma and recovery from it (Raghavan & Sandanapitchai 2019). Clauss-Ehlers (2004) uses the term "cultural resilience" to express how cultural values, language, customs, and norms can be used to fortify oneself against adversity. Examining the cultural supports that work as protective factors in creating children's resilience will help you focus on what builds resilience rather than what chips away at it.

In addition to cultural supports that encourage the development of resilience, some children are more resilient than others due to temperament and factors such as caregiver–infant attachment. But for the most part, children's resilience skills need to be nurtured and supported. As trauma pioneer Bruce Perry reminds us, "Resilient children are made, not born" (Grogan 2013).

The good news is that the number one way of fostering resilience in children is also the number one activity you should be doing anyway. According to the Center on the Developing Child at Harvard University (n.d. c), "The single most common factor for children who develop resilience is at least one stable and committed relationship with a supportive parent, caregiver, or other adult." You can be that person for the children in your program. Chapter 6 delves into building relationships with children.

In addition to forming a strong positive relationship with children, teachers can help children develop these critical skills to boost their resilience (Pearson & Hall 2017; Reivich & Shatté 2002):

1. Emotional regulation—the ability to keep emotions in check and not be overwhelmed by feelings

2. Impulse control—the ability to stop and choose whether to act on a desire to do something or to delay gratification

3. Causal analysis—the ability to analyze and accurately decide what caused the problem being faced

4. Realistic optimism—the ability to maintain a positive thinking style without ignoring real-life constraints

5. Empathy—the ability to understand the feelings and needs of others

6. Self-efficacy—the belief in one's own abilities to succeed and make a difference in the world

7. Reaching out—the ability to learn from mistakes and take on new opportunities

Many of these skills are explored further in the guiding principles that follow. By working one-on-one with each child, you can foster resilience that will predispose children to both recover from trauma and be ready to learn and succeed.

Principle 5: Help Children Learn to Regulate Their Emotions

According to resilience researcher Andrew Shatté, emotional regulation is the most important ability associated with resilience (Pearson & Hall 2017). Children who have experienced trauma may be easily triggered by sounds, smells, sights, and misconstrued words and actions into a fight-flight-freeze reactive mode (National Center on Safe Supportive Learning Environments, n.d.). At these times, their stress hormone levels increase and survival becomes their focus. Learning is put on hold when body and brain are on alert (Center on the Developing Child, n.d. e). Your primary focus is on how to turn this situation around.

One major part of your strategy should concentrate on setting up the program environment to reduce triggers. Chapter 5 provides guidance on how to design a space and plan a schedule to make children feel safe and comfortable. When triggers do arise for a child—perhaps a backfiring car sounds like a gunshot or a thunderstorm brings back memories of flooding—use a two-step approach: first, help children calm down, and second, when their stress has been reduced, help them learn how to regulate their emotions. By doing so, you open children up to a chance to focus on learning: "Children who have experienced adversities but demonstrate adaptive behaviors, such as the ability to manage their emotions, are more likely to have positive outcomes" (Murphey & Sacks 2018, 10).

When children are overwrought, angry, and acting out, go with them to the calming area in your classroom (see Chapter 5). Help the child release the intense feelings by squeezing balls and other pliable toys, playing with sensory materials, doing deep breathing exercises, reading books about characters who have similar emotions, listening and moving to music, or rocking tenderly with you.

You might also try what are known as mental "hookups"—physical exercises designed specifically to help children calm down during meltdowns or periods of high anxiety (see Fig. 5). You can do this by having a child stand with their legs and arms crossed in front of their body. The child places the palms of their hands against each other, with the fingers interlocked. Then ask the child to loop their hands underneath their arms in a pretzel fashion and hold that position for as long as they can, with two to five minutes being the ideal. This exercise uses movement to refocus the brain's activity and help the child calm themselves (Integrated Learning Strategies 2017).

When children have calmed, they are ready to learn some ways to regulate their emotions. Emotional regulation involves both cognitive and psychological processes, including becoming aware of one's feelings, learning the difference between emotional states, tolerating feelings without fear of losing control and expressing them safely, and moving from co-regulation with the help of an adult to self-regulation (Craig 2008).

Remember that emotional regulation is a skill, and like all skills, it takes continuing practice to be learned and mastered. Here are some ways you can work on emotional regulation with children:

> Be a role model always. Talk calmly, quietly, and warmly, sometimes known as "low and slow." Share your own feelings and what you do to keep them under control with children. Your calming behavior can be contagious to children who are dysregulated.

> Use feeling charts to help children learn to identify and label feelings. Charts can be easily made using emoticons or photographs of children in the program posing to represent a variety of feelings.

> Encourage children to make drawings, paintings, or collages of faces to illustrate different feelings, noting how colors can be used to express emotions.

> Provide children with ideas for different activities they can do to deal with a feeling they are experiencing. For example, if they feel scared, they can talk with a teacher about it and plan for how to address their fear. They could also cuddle up with a stuffed animal and a blanket on a beanbag chair for comfort, act out what has scared them in dramatic play, or focus on something fun that will take their mind in a different direction, such as playing outside on the slide with a friend.

> Use books about feelings to give children the vocabulary they need to describe their emotions. Go beyond basic labels like happy and sad—identify

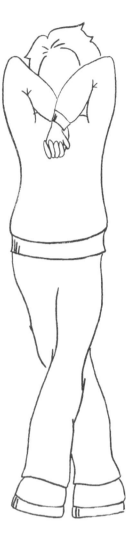

Figure 5. Using the hookup move to self-calm.

emotions and facial expressions as delighted, thrilled, or cheery. This builds vocabulary and teaches synonyms, and it helps children learn to identify the nuances of emotions.

> Teach children to take notice of how their body feels and how to put those feelings into words: "I see that your hands are in fists. I wonder how you are feeling inside that made you tighten your hands like that."

> Offer sensory activities like sand play, water play, and finger painting every day for children to work through emotions. Provide soothing natural materials to explore.

> Take children outdoors every day where they can exercise and use their large muscles and loud voices.

> Encourage dramatic play so children can express emotions and work through their fears by role playing. If a child needs help regulating emotions, occasionally enter the play: "I hear you yelling at the baby doll because she won't stop crying. That must be very frustrating that she won't stop. I wonder what else you could try to help her calm down."

> Put on skits and puppet shows and use persona dolls (dolls given a particular identity and treated as classmates and friends who often invite children to help solve a problem) to act out the main characters expressing their emotions acceptably.

> Help children problem solve and reframe frustrated thinking: "It's hard to wait for snack time when we're hungry. What can we make for our afternoon snack that we will be able to eat right away without having to wait to warm it up?"

> Encourage children to use self-talk to calm themselves down and to manage challenges: "When I get discouraged or worried, sometimes I give myself pep talks in my head. I tell myself, 'I'm really good at drawing. I bet I can make beautiful roses on this cake out of icing.' I wonder if that would help you."

> Help children use tools to keep their emotions in check, such as deep breathing, yoga poses, and visualization techniques.

> Display a "Cooling Off" poster with words and photos that convey strategies for regulating feelings. Some suggestions might be drawing, listening to calm music, shaking a glitter jar (see Appendix 3), walking with an adult, taking a deep belly breath, and crumpling paper and tossing it in a basket (Nicholson, Perez, & Kurtz 2019). Near the poster, place materials in a basket that correspond to some of the strategies.

As children gradually move from co-regulating with your assistance to self-regulating, they are less likely to be ruled by their emotions and can better maintain a state of being present.

Principle 6: Use Positive Guidance When Dealing with Children's Challenging Behaviors

Let's cut to the chase: Punishment, suspension, and expulsion are inappropriate for *any* young child. While the symptoms and behaviors that typically accompany experiencing trauma can challenge the patience of any educator, it is vital to always keep in mind that children are not trying to grate on your nerves or to intentionally misbehave. They are dealing with fears, and their brains are in survival mode. This state leads many children to act out in ways that disturb others. Take, for example, Hugh:

Hugh's mother has been addicted to drugs since before Hugh's birth. A neighbor continually complained to authorities that 5-year-old Hugh was being left alone. Nothing happened until a few months ago when Hugh found some matches and started a fire big enough for the fire department to have to come and extinguish it. Fortunately, no one was hurt, but Hugh was removed from his home and placed in foster care. He is quiet and withdrawn at his new foster home, barely speaking even when asked a question. At preschool, however, he pushes others when they are in his way, tells other children what to do, and demands that things be done his way.

Ms. Stafford, his preschool teacher, has tried several techniques to address the behaviors, starting with positive reinforcement for good behaviors. This technique has worked well with many other children. Disappointed when this brings no change in Hugh's behavior, she tries scolding, taking away privileges, shaming (for keeping everyone from being able to eat lunch because Hugh won't take a seat), and ignoring (when Hugh starts yelling and throwing things outside). Not wanting to resort to more severe punishments when those approaches don't work, Ms. Stafford talks the situation over with colleagues and becomes convinced that the solution to Hugh's aggressive behavior is to put Hugh in time-out and have him reflect on his behavior.

In time-out, however, Hugh sits in the chair and holds onto its sides and jumps with the chair. Thinking Hugh will eventually tire of this behavior, Ms. Stafford assigns Hugh to time-out for most the day. In a test of wills, neither Ms. Stafford nor Hugh will relent.

Ms. Stafford is now at her wit's end. Her traditional approach to guidance has had no effect on Hugh's challenging behaviors other than to escalate them. Hugh's behavior and outlook are deteriorating, and Ms. Stafford is out of ideas and patience.

Ms. Stafford believes that Hugh is intentionally misbehaving. She fails to understand that Hugh is in reaction mode. His brain is in a fight-flight-freeze frame of mind, seeking survival. Putting Hugh in time-out triggers his feelings of abandonment and not being cared about. Moreover, it does nothing to help Hugh regulate his emotions. As experts on trauma-sensitive care have noted, "Time-outs will be terrifying to children with trauma histories. Being abandoned and sent away as a punishment will be more triggering" (Nicholson, Perez, & Kurtz 2019, 161).

Time-out, zero-tolerance policies, and other punitive discipline techniques have little effect on changing the behavior of any child. For children like Hugh, they can have the additional ill effect of retraumatizing the child and sending the child a message that they are unlikeable. Ms. Stafford must help Hugh regulate his emotions in a safe place. Until he is calm and can release his fear, Hugh will have difficulty focusing on learning and interacting with others in positive ways. To this end, Ms. Stafford might try some of the following techniques (Downing 2016; Jennings 2019b; Nicholson, Perez, & Kurtz 2019):

> Rather than time-out, offer Hugh "time-in." This is an invitation for a child and teacher to sit together and connect. It enables children to feel safe and in control—factors that have been missing from Hugh's life.

> Speak calmly and in a lowered voice when Hugh pushes a child or throws a chair or blocks. "Hugh, I can see that you are upset, but I can't let you throw things or hurt anyone. Let's go to the calming corner. You can throw beanbags or squeeze the squishy balls to get rid of your unhappy feelings. I'm going to sit there with you until you're feeling better."

> Refrain from asking Hugh to explain his behavior by asking questions like "Why did you jump in the chair? Couldn't you at least have sat still in time-out?" Hugh may be just as puzzled by the way he acts as Ms. Stafford is. Children with a history of trauma (and most young children in general) have little self-knowledge or understanding of *why* they behave as they do.

> Acknowledge Hugh's feelings: "I can see that you're getting frustrated with the puzzle. I get that way at times, too. You might enjoy doing the one with fruit instead. I know that you like bananas and grapes a lot."

> Offer Hugh choices (all of which are acceptable to Ms. Stafford) so that he gains a sense of control: "Hugh, would you rather squeeze one of the stress balls or read a book with me?" When he is calm, the teacher could even offer Hugh choices regarding his behavior when it has been out of control: "Hugh, when you had an outburst this morning, you were very upset, and so was I. Let's think of some things you might do to help you calm down when you feel this way." This approach gives Hugh some control over his behavior without making him explain why this behavior occurred.

> Let Hugh know what he should be doing rather than what he shouldn't be doing: "Hugh, I'd like you to come sit at the lunch table next to me" rather than "Hugh, we're all hungry and you're wasting everyone's time by just standing there."

> Offer Hugh and all children an opportunity to participate in making classroom rules. Children are more likely to buy in and follow the rules when they have had a say in developing them: "Everyone, Hugh is suggesting that we need a rule that if we want to run, we need to do it outside.

Who Gets Expelled?

As far back as 2005, researcher Walter Gilliam found that preschoolers were being expelled at a rate three times higher than were children in grades K–12. For children enrolled in non-state-run pre-K programs, the rate was 13 times higher than in K–12 (Gilliam 2005).

Today, the rate of expulsion remains unacceptably high—more than 5,000 pre-K children are expelled each year (Council for Professional Recognition 2019). This translates into roughly 250 preschool children being suspended or expelled every single day (Malik 2017).

Hugh's behavior in the program, and Ms. Stafford's frustration at not being able to successfully address it, puts him at risk of being suspended or expelled. Being male puts him at an even greater risk: Boys compose 54 percent of the preschool population, yet 79 percent of preschool suspensions happen to boys. Moreover, boys represent 82 percent of children suspended multiple times (US Department of Education Office for Civil Rights 2014).

If Hugh had a disability, the odds of suspension or expulsion would likewise increase. Students with disabilities receive twice as many of these disciplinary actions as do their peers without disabilities (US Department of Education Office for Civil Rights 2014).

And if Hugh were Black, Latino, or Native American, the likelihood of his suspension or expulsion would go up even more. Black children are suspended or expelled at 3.2 times the rate of White children. Native American children have a rate 2 times that of their White counterparts, and Latino children are suspended or expelled 1.3 times as often as White children (Owens & McLanahan 2019).

Part of the reason for the discrepancy in treatment is that schools serving children of color and children from low-income families are more likely than other schools to adopt zero-tolerance policies toward children's misbehaviors (Welch & Payne 2010). In these schools, even minor infractions can lead to punishments such as immediate suspension or expulsion.

But beyond this, there is documented differential treatment in the way preschool teachers and administrators treat children of different races. A Yale Child Center study found that educators of all races spend more time watching Black youngsters for disruptive behaviors than they do their White classmates (Wright 2020). Black boys in particular are at the receiving end of teachers' expectations of problem behaviors. They are given harsher disciplinary actions than are White boys exhibiting the same behaviors (Gilliam et al. 2016). Among all races, Black teachers hold the highest standards for Black boys' behavior (Mwenelupembe 2020).

These punitive practices serve no one—least of all the children. Expelled preschool children are more likely to be unprepared when they enter formal schooling in kindergarten. This negative impact carries on throughout their school careers, including a higher risk for school failure (Council for Professional Recognition 2019).

What do you think? That would mean that indoors we walk or sit or lie down, but we won't run."

> Let Hugh know that you have positive expectations that he will be following the classroom rules. "Hugh, I know that you'll be able to put the blocks on the shelf when you're done playing with them. Thank you."

> Choose words that de-escalate tensions, such as "I wonder if . . ." or "Let's try . . ." or "Suppose we . . ." or "I wonder if we moved the easel outside if you'd enjoy painting where there's more space. I bet the fresh air will feel good, too."

> Credit Hugh publicly whenever it is appropriate to do so: "Thank you for bringing over the book so that I can read it to you and Tessa. That was very thoughtful of you, Hugh." If the teacher needs to call attention to negative behavior, however, she should do it privately by calling Hugh over to a place away from the others, having him sit him down, and quietly telling him, "Hugh, you know that we have a rule that you can't throw things. In fact, you helped make this rule. You might have hit someone when you threw that block. My job is to keep everyone in this classroom safe—including you."

If Ms. Stafford were to continue to treat Hugh's outbursts as misbehavior rather than as symptoms of a deeper problem, the result for Hugh would very likely be suspension or even expulsion from preschool. Children like Hugh, who are not being responded to with social and emotional support, try educators' patience and all too often the only recourse seems to be removing the child from the program (see "Who Gets Expelled?").

While suspension and expulsion are a disservice to any child, for the traumatized child, it can do irreversible damage. Expulsion is another form of trauma. It only serves to reinforce for children that they are not wanted, destroying any relationship that may have been formed with their teacher. Rather than remediate the situation, it sets children back even further. Suspension and expulsion ought never be regarded as a possibility for young children.

Principle 7: Be a Role Model to Children on How to Act and Approach Learning

Teachers and parents have the power to influence what children think, feel, and do. If you like singing "Head, Shoulders, Knees, and Toes," reading *Pete the Cat* books, and making homemade granola for snacks, those will be the favorites of many of the children. They look to you for guidance, inspiration, and validation—and for assistance in maneuvering the complexities of life.

By following your lead, children can begin to heal from trauma and become engaged learners. Think about how you might model the following and use these activities to help children grow and learn:

> How to use the indoor and outdoor spaces to play independently or with a friend, a small group, or the whole group

> How to read books, write, and count

> How to appreciate nature, garden, and nurture pets

> How to create art and music and how to dance

> How to make, maintain, and support friendships

> How to attentively listen to others

> How to self-calm and self-regulate

> How to build on people's strengths, not their weaknesses or failings

> How to be realistically optimistic

> How to listen and react with empathy

> How to be kind and grateful

> How to solve problems

> How to learn from failures

> How to use positive self-talk as a resilience technique

> How to laugh, enjoy oneself, and have fun while learning

Principle 8: Help Children Turn Negative Thinking Around

Many children who have experienced trauma have had to deal with great negativity in their lives. This can lead children to act in unpleasant ways, making them difficult to be around. Children who have experienced trauma may misinterpret others' actions and attribute negative intent when there is none. They may focus on their own pessimistic thoughts. For many children who have experienced trauma, life feels like an ongoing worst-case scenario.

A key strategy in building resilience in young children is for them to develop thinking that is realistically optimistic. You can do this with children by gently disputing their negative thinking and showing them when it's not rooted in fact.

Optimism can be learned, no matter how innately pessimistic a person may be or how negative their life circumstances have been (Seligman 2005). By going through what has been dubbed the ABCDE model, educators can help children as young as 2½ learn to reframe their negative thinking to be positive (Hall & Pearson 2004). Here's how the model works (based on Colker & Koralek 2019 and Seligman 2005):

A = an **adverse event**

For the purposes of this example, the teacher, Ms. Jones, asks 4-year-old Oliver to leave the sand table and find a new place to play.

B = **beliefs** and thoughts about the adverse event

Oliver reads into the request and takes it as a command, which is triggering for him. His teacher takes away the choice he had in deciding to play at the sand table, which makes him feel like he has no control. He interprets his teacher's behavior as being punishing and targeted at him. He feels that Ms. Jones clearly doesn't like him.

C = the **consequences** of having these thoughts and beliefs

Oliver goes into survival mode and gets very angry. He throws a bunch of props into the sand table, nearly hitting some children playing there, and shouts at Ms. Jones, "You're being mean. You're always mean to me. I hate it here. You like everyone but me."

Ms. Jones asks Oliver to accompany her to the calming corner: "Oliver, I can see that you are very upset. Let's go to the calming corner together. Why don't you throw some sensory balls at the target or hit a punching doll, if you prefer. That will help you get rid of some of these feelings that are so strong. Afterward, when you feel a bit calmer, we can talk."

Once Oliver gets more control over his emotions, Ms. Jones sits facing Oliver on beanbag chairs, and continues with the model.

D = **disputation** of the pessimistic beliefs

Ms. Jones begins by calmly explaining why she asked Oliver to leave the sand play area: "I am sorry that you thought I was mean. That was most certainly not my intent. The problem was that there were too many children at the sand table. It was getting too crowded for everyone to safely play there. You were the first to arrive there, so I asked you to move on because other children did not have such a long turn."

Ms. Jones also disputes Oliver's interpretation that she didn't like him by recalling many times when she demonstrated her positive feelings toward him. "At lunch today I asked you to help set the tables with me. Yesterday, after you fell off your trike, I cleaned the scrape and gave you a big hug. And last week at group time, I asked you to sit next to me and help take attendance. Can you think about how you felt at these times? I hope you know that I like you a lot."

After Oliver reflects on Ms. Jones's words, he nods and admits that those were nice times.

> E = **energization** from successfully disputing the negative thoughts and realizing that the situation is not as feared
>
> Oliver feels better about his relationship with Ms. Jones and why she asked him to leave the sand table. Now he doesn't mind leaving and asks Ms. Jones if they can read a book together in the library center.

Obviously, it will take more than a one-time conversation like the one Ms. Jones had with Oliver to change his negative thinking. Using the ABCDE process repeatedly and regularly will help children like Oliver who tend to instinctively think negatively to develop a positive thinking style. Each time you hear a child expressing their negative thinking, take the opportunity to help the child regulate their emotions and then help them reframe their negative thinking in a positive way.

For some children, learning to self-regulate emotions and dispute negative thoughts is a straightforward process. For others whose negative thinking runs deep, it will take considerable time. As always, be patient.

One final point about the above example: Ms. Jones should examine her own thinking for possible bias toward Oliver. Is there some truth to Oliver's assertion that she doesn't like him? How might his challenging behavior be consciously or unconsciously affecting how she interacts with him?

Turning children's negative thinking into optimism offers profound benefits. Optimists, as compared to pessimists, are healthier, live an average of nine years longer than pessimists, and have happier, more fulfilling lives (Colker & Koralek 2019). Optimism is correlated with self-efficacy, problem-solving skills, and the ability to learn from mistakes (Seligman 2007). These are the same skills that children exposed to trauma often lack and need so they can prosper in preschool and kindergarten.

Principle 9: Enrich Children's Lives with Art, Music, and Dance

All people need art to have a fulfilling life. Art enriches the soul and brings beauty to life. Here is what Sir Philip Pullman (ALMA, n.d.), award-winning British novelist, says:

> Children need art and stories and poems and music as much as they need love and food and fresh air and play. If you don't give a child food, the damage quickly becomes visible. If you don't let a child have fresh air and play, the damage is also visible, but not so quickly. If you don't give a child love, the damage might not be seen for some years, but it's permanent.
>
> But if you don't give a child art and stories and poems and music, the damage is not so easy to see. It's there, though. . . . That hunger exists in many children, and often it is never satisfied because it has never been awakened. Many children in every part of the world are starved for something that feeds and nourishes their soul in a way that nothing else ever could or ever would.

Beyond the cultural value art brings to children's lives, it also serves a major educational and therapeutic value. Children communicate through their artwork, music, dance, and movement. For many children, it is easier to express their emotions through these avenues than it is through talking. For children with a history of trauma who may not comprehend what has happened to them and are not always aware of what their feelings are—let alone why they feel the way they do—the arts may be the best way of giving them a voice. Engaging in arts also offers restorative powers for children who have experienced trauma (Sorrels 2015). The rhythm of music, for instance, can help organize a brain that is disorganized (Baker 2007).

The arts are a prime outlet for communicating about the trauma. Drawing, painting, modeling with clay, dancing, singing, and moving to music offer a path to survival and recovery. Listen to and observe children as they create and work through their emotions in art; let the information you gain guide your next steps.

Provide children materials, space, and time for creating, moving, and expressing themselves each day, not just for special projects. Art, music, and dance should also be taken outdoors. Singing with children at arrival and departure times or during cleanup or transitions becomes a ritual that gives children a sense of belonging and security.

Principle 10: Look Beyond Children's Traumas and Celebrate the Joys in Life

Throughout this book there is a global theme: Your knowledge, skills, and dedication will help children experiencing trauma to heal and flourish. It's easy to get caught up in the many challenges that must be faced to help children get to the point where they will heal.

Healing, though, is just part of the goal. What about the flourishing part? Children who have been traumatized are children first, and they are due the same aspirations and high expectations that every child in your program is due. Helping children flourish means taking a deep breath and refocusing on the lightness and laughter that is, happily, also a part of teaching.

Help children find activities and experiences that let them feel good about themselves and their place in the world. If a child loves music, use that as a forum for the child to shine. The patterning in music can be used as a springboard for developing math skills. If a child is good at throwing and catching balls, incorporate physical activity as a part of learning. Have them make up part of a continuing story as the ball is thrown and caught. Let their strengths and interests guide the presentation of content.

Encourage children to be creative and silly and to delight in a belly laugh when something humorous happens. As noted previously, one of the chief goals of a healing-centered program is that children be able to share in the normalcy of childhood. This means that all children deserve high-quality programming, nurturing interactions, a warm atmosphere, and an environment where they can be curious and explore, experiment, and discover with competence and confidence.

You also want to help children look beyond themselves and develop empathy and kindness toward others. Consider having a gratitude box prominently displayed in your room (Colker & Koralek 2019). Each day have the children think of something good that happened for which they are grateful and would like to share with others. A gratitude memory can be anything from "My teacher picked me to help get out the cots for rest time" to "They served chicken fingers for lunch" to "I made a pretty collage." At a designated time, help the children write their memories on index cards that can be inserted in the gratitude box. The children can illustrate the cards and sign them or leave them unsigned. Don't forget to write and insert your own gratitude card. At a morning meeting perhaps once a week, randomly pick out a card from the gratitude box and read it aloud to the group. If the card has been signed, have the author—even if it should be you—tell the group how this memory made them feel. If unsigned, have the group talk about that gratitude memory together.

Taking the time to reflect on and express gratitude not only makes children kinder but also counteracts the trauma-related effects of stress and depression in the one who is grateful (Colker & Koralek 2019; Seligman 2005). By looking beyond themselves, children feel better.

Activities like this will also make children who have experienced trauma feel both like they are a part of the group and that they are moving beyond the trauma into a world where their trauma no longer defines who they are and what they can do. You want children to be able to embrace joy and feel that the world can be a good and loving place.

Principle 11: Remember that You Don't Have to Have All the Answers

The most knowledgeable and confident people know their limitations and willingly admit to the need to learn more. You are not expected to know everything. If you don't have the training or experience to know how best to respond, seek advice. This is nothing to chastise yourself for. To the contrary, you should be proud of yourself for doing what is best for children.

If you don't know how to handle a child's challenging behavior or how to prevent other children from shunning a traumatized child who is being obnoxious to them, ask your administrator or a counselor or specialist for guidance and support. They can help strategize how to help a child who bites or to stop bullying in its tracks.

Likewise, don't feel you have to be certain before referring a child to a mental health, special education, or counseling professional for evaluation. Together with the specialist and the child's family, decide if the child could benefit from some type of intervention.

Depending on the need, there will be many times you will want to consult with the child's family or guardians. If it is a policy question, check with your administrator.

Your colleagues can also offer helpful information. Often you need to check with specialists. If the child is seeing a therapist, that person may have the answer you are seeking, although be prepared if this person cannot answer anything personal about the child due to doctor–patient confidentiality. If you are part of a school system, there is often a psychologist or special educator on staff who can assist you.

The point is that you are not alone during any of this. You are in the front line, but you are also part of a trained and prepared program and community that are there to support you—just as you support children. With patience and dedication, you can turn children's fears and insecurities around.

A Path Forward

Children with a trauma history need and deserve to be viewed, educated, and treated as children first, not as trauma victims. This means that they too can share in the educational future you envision for the children in your program. By using the guiding principles presented in this chapter, you can steer children with a traumatic past toward a present and future with promise. The next few chapters offer further guidance on how you might best do this.

CHAPTER Five

Establishing a Safe and Inviting Environment for Learning

The physical environment sets the tone for all that goes on in your program. It is the key factor in setting the stage for implementing the curriculum and, when designed with the needs of all children in mind, enables children to feel safe and valued so that they can learn and thrive. Looking at your environment through the eyes of a child who has experienced trauma can give you new insights as to how to best design and use your environment to promote healing.

In addition, because the physical environment can either affirm or suppress children's identities, it is critical to use materials and furnishings that support all children's cultures, races, needs, and interests. However unintentional it may be, the program environment can itself be a form of racial microaggression (Sue et al. 2007). If, for example, the books on display, the music that is available to listen to, or the food choices offered reflect the cultures of only some of the children, families, and staff, some will feel that they are not a part of the learning community.

According to the Reggio Emilia approach, there are three teachers in the life of a child: the parent, the teacher, and the environment. The environment represents a program's values about children and should reflect the belief that children have a right to learn in beautiful spaces designed with their needs in mind (Biermeier 2015). This philosophy applies to all children, particularly those who have endured trauma. Whether or not your program follows the Reggio Emilia approach, the physical environment is a critical component.

The way you design your space can make children feel good about themselves and learning. You establish an environment that makes children feel secure, respected, and valued through

> Arranging the physical space for exploring and learning

> Providing developmentally appropriate toys, materials, and equipment, including a calming area where children can regulate their emotions and books that will help children heal and learn

> Establishing a program structure that brings order and predictability to the day

Design a Physical Environment That Supports Children's Emotional, Social, Physical, and Learning Needs

As you set up a healing-centered environment, be sure that the children who work and play there are picking up messages that reflect your teaching goals. Strive to have an environment where children feel the following:

> I am safe.

> I am valued.

> I belong.

> People care about and support me.

> I can do things on my own.

> I can make and play with friends.

> There are interesting things to learn.

> I can be my authentic self and explore my identity.

> My background and identity are respected.

> I can calm myself down when I'm upset.

> I can make choices.

> I can make mistakes.

> This is a place that encourages hope and optimism.

> This is a fun place to be.

How you set up the space and encourage children to use it tells them what their time at the program will be like. For example, if there are large open spaces where children can run around and get in each other's way, children are likely to perceive this to be a place where they might get hurt, where chaos rules, and where there is the same unpredictability that often comes with trauma. Conversely, if the space is arranged so that children can play safely, choose and return materials on their own, and move around without knocking into furniture or other people, children are more likely to feel that this is a safe place they can explore.

When you arrange the environment, try getting down to the children's height so you can adjust furniture and materials to match the children's perspective. "Environmental Supports for Children with a History of Trauma," on pages 42–43, offers suggestions for designing your program's environment. These will support all the children you teach, but special thought has been given to making the environment responsive to children with a history of trauma.

Provide Materials and Equipment that Support Learning and Healing

Selecting toys, materials, and equipment to support children who have experienced trauma starts with the same developmentally appropriate principles for all early childhood programs. Ensure that all children's cultures and languages are represented in books, recipe cards, play foods and utensils, music and musical instruments, dramatic play clothing, and prop boxes. Understand where each child is developmentally and provide materials that allow them to experience success and also be challenged to learn new skills and concepts. Keep in mind that children with a trauma history may not be at the same developmental level as many other children their age. Also, materials and equipment must be safe for children's use and should encourage each child to explore, experiment, take risks, be creative, and solve problems.

Not all materials need to be purchased. With help from the children's families, you can make musical instruments, cardboard blocks, games, puppets, flannel boards, prop boxes for dramatic play, and many other materials and props. Doing so makes for fun, rewarding projects and helps keep costs down.

As you put together your inventory, focus on two special categories of materials that support children who have experienced trauma. The first group of materials is for a calming area. The second is for your book or library center.

Provide a Calming Center

While each component of the environment is important, children who have lived with trauma benefit from having an area where they can go to calm down when they are in a reactive mode. While in a fight-flight-freeze state, children cannot focus or listen to anyone trying to interact with them. They need a sensory break to de-escalate their fears and regulate the emotions that are overwhelming their brains.

When children are in this state, they typically feel like running away or hiding in a corner. Provide a safe haven for them—a nook, a corner area, a loft, or any place away from noisy areas with a lot of action, such as the block and water play areas. Some teachers like to enclose the space by putting up a tent or a beach umbrella or suspending mosquito netting from the ceiling. Give the space a name, like "cozy corner," "calming center," "peace place," or "cool-down corner." The important thing is that this space be dedicated to this one purpose and that children are aware of and encouraged to go there whenever they need to decompress.

Environmental Supports for Children with a History of Trauma

Environmental Feature	How this Supports Children Who Have Experienced Trauma
The inside and outside areas are free of health and physical dangers, allowing children to explore and experiment.	Children gain a sense of safety and security when they can play with enthusiasm without fear of being harmed.
There is a welcoming area where families drop off and pick up children, communicate with educators, and find parenting and program resources.	Children are comforted and have less separation anxiety when their family members help transition them to and from the program.
Walls and furnishings are painted in neutral colors, and natural materials are used throughout.	Neutral colors and spaces promote calming and healing. Brain research shows that it is difficult for children to visually process a multitude of colors and stay on task (Dionne-Dostie et al. 2015). Bright colors may trigger the fight-flight-freeze response in children with a history of trauma.
When possible, natural lighting is used rather than fluorescent lights. When needed, soft floor lighting in corners of the room is turned on. Filters are used to minimize the harshness of fluorescent lights.	Bright lights are triggering for many children. Too much lighting can cause overstimulation and distractions (Vasandani 2015).
Bathrooms have child-size toilets and sinks, and handwashing materials are accessible.	Children take care of their own needs on their own schedules when bathrooms are designed for independent use. The experience of using the bathroom as a group can be triggering to some children and works against self-regulation.
Areas of the room are devoted to sensory exploration, such as sand and water tables, playdough and clays, and finger painting.	Children under stress need to self-regulate so they can pay attention and learn. Sensory play helps children become calm, work through emotions, and gain a sense of control over their environment.
Photographs of children and families are prominently displayed in cubbies, on room dividers, in the daily schedule, and in albums of field trips and home visits. There is an "All About Me" book for each child in the library center.	Photos reinforce a sense of belonging and comfort, especially for children who are feeling the pangs of separation. Seeing photos of themselves makes children feel appreciated as individuals and as members of a diverse learning community.
The room is neat and uncluttered. Displays are organized and appealing to the eye.	Overcrowded walls are distracting and negatively affect children's abilities to focus and learn (Association for Psychological Science 2014). Organized displays support a calming, less triggering environment and avoid overstimulating children's sensory systems.

Environmental Feature	How this Supports Children Who Have Experienced Trauma
In center-based programs, nap or rest time takes place in the classroom, with cots or mats placed where the children prefer. In both center-based and family child care programs, night lights are available. Adults stay close by.	Choices about where to nap and whether to have a light give children control of the situation, provide security, and reduce the chances of bad memories being triggered.
Self-serve snacks are available when children arrive and after nap or rest time. Children follow written and picture directions and sign their names on a sheet so teachers know who has eaten.	Making snacks self-serve puts children in control of their needs by letting them decide when they want to eat. Self-serving avoids stigmatizing children who come to the program not having eaten and supports independence and learning. Time is used more efficiently, allowing children more time to play in centers.

Set up the area to be welcoming. Use soft lighting. Stock the area with manipulatives and materials you feel will enable children to get out strong feelings and unwind, like these:

> Beanbag chairs, pillows, or floor cushions

> Rocking chair

> Blankets, afghans, throws, or a sleeping bag

> Fish tank with fish

> Beanbags and a hoop or other target

> Squishy manipulatives and balls

> Inflatable punching bags or punching balls

> Paper for crumpling and a trash can

> Bubbles

> Playdough or clay

> Sand tray

> Water play tub

> Kaleidoscopes

> Picture books on feelings and calming down

> Feelings charts that build emotional vocabulary (see Chapter 4)

> Headphones with classical or New Age music

> Bottle labeled "Calm-Down Lotion" filled with soothing body lotion

If space is at a premium and you do not have the room to create a separate area devoted to calming down, collect items in a calming basket that you can offer to children in a quiet area of the program. Stock the basket with items such as stress balls, playdough, books on feelings, squishy manipulatives, and kaleidoscopes.

Search for directions online for making calm-down bottles that can be put in a basket or your cozy corner. For example, paper clips and water can be added to a clear bottle. A magnetic wand moving on the jar's outside surface can then be used to drag the paper clips around. Or just add water and ocean-colored water beads to make a soothing, calming bottle. Anything that distracts children from the emotions that overwhelm them and allows them to breathe deeply and relax is helpful. (As referenced in Chapter 4, detailed information on creating a glitter jar to calm children appears in Appendix 3. This handout is intended to be shared with families, but you can make a glitter jar for your calming area too.)

Choose Books that Will Benefit Children with Trauma Experience

Bibliotherapy is a creative arts therapy that involves storytelling and reading specific texts with the purpose of healing. It is used in many contexts in early childhood education but is especially powerful as a tool to teach social and emotional skills. Because these skills are at the core of what children exposed to trauma need to come to terms with what they have experienced, reading and re-creating stories from picture books makes bibliotherapy especially effective.

By supplementing your existing book selection with titles that specifically address dealing with trauma and learning to regulate feelings, you can help children work through their emotions emanating from trauma. Other children without a trauma background will no doubt be drawn to having you read these books, too. But for children with a trauma history, they can be a much-needed tool for healing.

Reading books together with children offers rich opportunities to connect with them. For this reason and because of the individual nature of most trauma, rather than always reading to the whole group or even a small group of children, read together with individual children as well.

If the child you are reading with is comfortable with closeness, sit together on a couch or beanbag chair, away from the activity of the group. The calming center is often an ideal location because of its ambience. For children who are averse to touch, sitting next to each other in child-size and adult-size rockers might work well.

Read and discuss a book you have chosen specifically for a child as you would any other time you read. Here are some general guidelines:

> Introduce the book and explain to the child why you picked this book. Look at the book cover with the child, pointing out the names of the author and illustrator.

> Read the book aloud all the way through without stopping to ask questions the first time you read the book together so that the whole story and the rhythm of the words come through. Depending on the child, ask them to turn the pages of the book as you read it aloud.

> Read the book together again, this time stopping to discuss the characters, what happened to them, how they reacted, and what choices they made.

> Tailor your questions to fit the story being read, the child's developmental level, and the type of social and emotional support the child needs. Use the following suggestions as a starting point for your own questions (Colker & Koralek 2019, 70):

   - What happened to _____ in the story?

   - How did this make _____ feel?

   - What do you suppose _____ was thinking inside their head when this happened?

   - What do you think the adults felt about what happened?

   - Did _____ do the right thing?

   - What would you have told _____ to do?

   - How could you make _____ feel better?

   - Would you have ended the story like this? If not, how would you have ended it?

> As you read, relate the story to the child's experiences, or as much as you know about them. While you don't want to probe for details about trauma, let the child know that they are not alone. Many children exposed to trauma feel just that.

> Let children know that being scared, angry, or sad; crying; or feeling however the main character felt is normal. So are other feelings they may be having.

> Highlight for the child, if this is a part of the story, that the bad event was not the main character's fault. Many children feel they are to blame for the experienced trauma, so reassurance that it had nothing to do with them is important.

> Review how the main character came to terms with what was happening in the story and talk about whether this plan would work for the child.

> Reread the story together with the child as many times as the child would like.

> Encourage the child to re-create the story in a puppet show or skit or through art.

> Reiterate for the child that you are there to talk about the story and the child's feelings at any time.

Sample Book Reading Experience: *A Terrible Thing Happened*

Five-year-old Tiffany's dad recently died by suicide. Her mother is still in shock, and her older sister refuses to talk about what happened. Tiffany has been having uncharacteristic bouts of anger, yelling at her classmates outdoors and refusing to play with her friends during center time. Frequently this behavior ends with Tiffany collapsing in tears. Ms. Seymour has been encouraging Tiffany to express her feelings through art and dramatic play, which has been helpful.

Today Ms. Seymour wants to try discussing *A Terrible Thing Happened* (by Margaret M. Holmes) with Tiffany, which she introduced to her yesterday. Ms. Seymour has carefully thought about some questions she might ask Tiffany as they reflect on the story (see below).

Ms. Seymour asks Tiffany to sit with her on the couch in the cozy corner while Mr. Edwards works with the other children in centers. Ms. Seymour sits close to Tiffany and tells her that she picked this book about Sherman Smith, a raccoon, because something very bad happened in his life, and she thinks Tiffany can understand how Sherman feels. Ms. Seymour points out the scratchy blackish thought balloon on the cover and asks Tiffany what she thinks Sherman is thinking in his head. "Something that's bad and mean," says Tiffany. "It does look kind of frightening," agrees Ms. Seymour.

Ms. Seymour gently asks Tiffany questions about the story, listens intently, and comments on the child's responses. Ms. Seymour points out how the adults in the book try to make Sherman feel better, helping him feel safe and reassuring him that he was not responsible for the terrible thing that happened.

Ms. Seymour asks Tiffany some of the following questions, taking her cue from Tiffany as to how much she can absorb at one time. The teacher plans to discuss the questions she doesn't get to today another time.

1. Why do you think Sherman didn't want to remember what happened? Has that ever happened to you?

2. Why do you think Sherman's plan of not thinking about what happened didn't work?

3. What do you think Sherman was thinking in his head when he got a tummy ache and he felt sad?

4. Why do you think Sherman was so angry all the time? Have you ever felt that way?

5. Why was it important for Ms. Maple to help Sherman think about his feelings? What do you think his head was telling him when he started to think about his feelings?

6. Do you have someone in your life like Ms. Maple you like to talk to? You know that Mr. Edwards and I are always here to talk with you whenever you'd like. We both care about you very much.

7. How did drawing pictures help Sherman feel better when he was angry? Do you feel better when you draw pictures when you are angry?

8. Why do you think Sherman was afraid that he caused the terrible thing? Do you think it was his fault? What would you tell Sherman to make him feel better?

9. Do you think Sherman will stay happy? What could he do to stay happy?

10. Did you like the end of the book? Do you think it was a good ending? If you were the author of the book, how would you have ended the story?

Many excellent picture books address the different kinds of traumas children may face. Appendix 2 has a suggested list, and your school or public librarian can also help you identify appropriate titles. Read to children often, especially when they choose to play in the library area or want be in the calming center. Strive to have a one-on-one reading session with each child by the end of each week. Group read-alouds of books about feelings or shared experiences like a recent hurricane can take place before lunch or at morning or closing meetings.

In addition to reading books on the trauma-related subjects included in Appendix 2, stock your library on related topics that the whole group might benefit from. These include books on dealing with strong emotions like anger, jealousy, disappointment, fear, and anxiety, such as *Don't Feed the Worry Bug* (by Andi Green), *What to Do When It's Not Fair: A Kid's Guide to Handling Envy and Jealousy* (by Jacqueline B. Toner and Claire A. B. Freeland), or *B is for Breathe: The ABCs of Coping with Fussy and Frustrating Feelings* (by Melissa Boyd).

Books on positive feelings and skills, such as gratitude, optimism, kindness, hopefulness, grit, mindfulness, and being peaceful also benefit all children. Look for books such as *Kindness Starts With You* (by Jacquelyn Stagg), *I Am Peace: A Book of Mindfulness* (by Susan Verde), or *Firenze's Light* (by Jessica Collaço).

Bring Structure to the Environment Through the Daily Schedule

As with the layout and design of the program environment, a daily schedule can give children the sense of security they crave. Life with trauma is often one of chaos and uncertainty. Knowing what will be happening at each point in the day and in what sequence offers children stability and a chance to recoup the normality of everyday life. As such, one of the most important things educators can do to help children who have experienced trauma is to create a daily schedule and review it each day with children.

Post the schedule on a wall or the back of a room divider at the children's eye level in a spot where they can consult it whenever they want and where you can discuss it with children together. You might point out to Bella, for example, that after the group comes in from outdoors, you will read aloud a story to everyone while the children serving as the day's helpers assist Mr. Richman in getting ready for lunch. Illustrate each item in the schedule with a picture. Some educators like using photos of the children in their program engaged in the various activities to illustrate the daily schedule. A sample daily schedule is shown on the following page.

While having a posted daily schedule promotes stability and predictability, there are some strategies you can incorporate into your daily schedule to further help children who have been traumatized. For instance, think about the following:

> Set a leisurely pace for the day's activities. Having to rush from one activity to the next doesn't allow children to become fully engaged in play. A hurried schedule also works against self-regulation.

> Build in attendance and a daily check-in with each child. Children might move a headshot of themselves with Velcro backing to an attendance chart each morning. Use this time to ask each child how they feel, how they slept, and if anything interesting has happened since they were last at the program.

Sample Daily Schedule for Preschool

 Arrival and Breakfast

 Morning Meeting and Attendance

 Choice Time in Centers

 Outdoor Choice Time

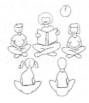 Storytime and Lunch Preparation

 Lunch

 Nap or Rest Time

 Choice Time

 Afternoon Meeting

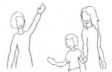 Departure

> Provide an hour or more of scheduled time each day for children to play and work in learning centers where they get to choose where they will be, what they will be working on, and with whom. This gives children a sense of control over their lives and the power to persevere in what they desire.

> Schedule an hour or more of outdoor play time daily where children choose what they will do and with whom. Exercising outdoors also helps children work through emotions, calm themselves, and refresh themselves for learning.

> Schedule time for children to both work on activities of their own design and follow structured activities. Children need both structure and choice to thrive.

> Schedule group meetings at the start and the end of the program day. To allay children's fears of unpredictability, preview the day at the morning meeting, highlighting activities on the daily schedule. At the end of the day, children can review how the day went and feel good about what they accomplished.

> Keep transitions to a minimum and build them into scheduled activities rather than making them separate items on the schedule. Transitions can be harrowing for children who have experienced trauma, as they involve going from the known to the unknown. Below are some of the ways you can make transitions less triggering for children with a trauma history:

  • Build cleanup into center time, giving children a five-minute warning. A sand timer will make this more concrete to children who do not yet understand time.

  • Turn other transitions into routines that have rituals. For example, play music, sing a song, ring a bell, or blow a harmonica to signal the start of a transition or to give a 5-minute warning.

  • Break the transition down into smaller steps when giving directions: "When you've finished eating, the first thing to do is stand up and push your chair in under the table. Then take your plate and throw the waste into the trash can. Afterward, put the empty plate on the pile."

  • Model the transition for children ahead of time, walking through each step.

  • Encourage families to send lovies (comfort objects) from home for the times children need a boost of emotional support. For instance, when it's time to stand in line to go to the library, let Sean get his plushy wolf out of his cubby and take it with him.

  • Place contact paper cutouts of feet on the floor to indicate where children should stand when lining up or sitting around tables. Children who need personal space will feel that it is being respected.

  • Stay close to children to offer emotional support and to assist them in activities such as putting coats on and taking them off, getting out mats for rest time, brushing their teeth, and toileting.

Because having a predictable schedule is so important to children exposed to trauma, if there are going to be changes to the schedule on a particular day, announce them ahead of time, if possible. Explain why there is a change and how it will affect the children's scheduled activities.

Tips for the Physical Environment

> **Remember that environments are not static.** Every group of children is different, with unique capabilities and needs that change and evolve over time. Observe how children play and work in the environment and adjust it to accommodate what you see. For example, you might rearrange furniture to more closely supervise children's play or provide more large motor activities indoors.

> **Be judicious in offering a choice of materials.** While having a choice of materials is extremely important to children with a trauma experience, having more than a few choices can become frustrating and even overwhelming. Be thoughtful and modest in putting out selections. Try displaying just a few high-interest items attractively on each shelf.

> **Rotate toys, materials, and equipment.** As children's needs and interests change, swap in new items to keep children engaged and learning. For example, offer manipulatives like beads, pegs, and collage materials to build on a child's rapidly developing fine motor skills. In addition, change materials to reflect the group's new areas of study and project work. If you are beginning an investigation on balls, for example, remove some of the materials from a prior study on insects and add balls and related items for children to explore both indoors and outdoors.

> **Give children your attention during choice time.** Because so much is required of educators, they sometimes look at choice time as opportunities to do paperwork, plan, or get caught up with colleagues, especially when outdoors. Children with a trauma background in particular need your attention during activities they have chosen to do. If you are in a center-based program, work with your supervisor, co-teacher, and other colleagues to figure out a way to have time for meaningful contact with each child. For example, bring in a parent volunteer to do a science experiment with a small group of children while you spend some individual time with a child. Or if you are in a school setting, a second grader might be thrilled to come in and read aloud to a few children. Another parent volunteer might be happy to do some paperwork tasks to free up your time.

Spending time with children during play is a prime opportunity to model and work with them on learning to regulate their emotions and make learning connections: "Kavya, you seem to really like playing with the maracas. Would you like us to both put on earphones so we can listen and shake along to the song 'Shake Your Maraca'?"

A Path Forward

Having a physical environment that supports children and makes them feel safe, valued, and important promotes recovery from trauma. Look at your setting through the eyes of the children you teach. Do they see themselves reflected there? Is it a safe and inviting place for them? Is this an environment where they can work through troubling emotions and also explore, experiment, solve problems, and learn?

Chapter 6 focuses on how the people in the environment—educators and children—can achieve the program's goals of healing and thriving through close connections with each other.

CHAPTER
Six | Connecting with Children

There is probably nothing more important in early childhood education and for human beings than relationships. Every child needs to feel connected to their teacher to feel secure enough to learn. When it comes to teaching young children, relationships must come before content.

For children with a history of trauma, positive relationships with teachers are crucial. Strong, caring relationships buffer children from traumatic stress and build their capacity for emotional and behavioral regulation (Lazar 2019). Educators inspire children and become a support network, which improves the likelihood of a positive future (Wright 2017). As noted in earlier chapters, building and maintaining a relationship with children is the most important thing you can do to promote children's resilience. A caring, nurturing relationship with a teacher has the power to prevent or reverse the toxic impact of trauma for young children.

An updated version of the classic book *The Boy Who Was Raised As a Dog: And Other Stories From a Child Psychiatrist's Notebook—What Traumatized Children Can Teach Us About Loss, Love, and Healing* (Perry & Szalavitz 2017) explores the importance of connections of any length, noting how even a brief connection can be therapeutic to a child who has experienced trauma:

> An attentive, attuned, and responsive person will help create opportunities for a traumatized child to control the dose and pattern of rewiring their trauma-related associations. . . . The more we can provide each other these moments of simple, human connection—even a brief nod or a moment of eye contact—the more we'll be able to heal those who have suffered traumatic experience. (308-9)

Forming these close connections is perhaps the greatest gift an educator can give to a child who has experienced trauma.

How to Foster Relationships When Children Have Experienced Trauma

Children who have been affected by trauma need to be assured that adults can keep them safe and secure and want to support them in all ways. Trauma expert Barbara Sorrels (2015, 163) writes, "Safety is not found in a place. Safety is first and foremost found in the context of a warm, nurturing, and protective relationship."

Researchers have identified three dimensions of teacher–student relationships: conflict, dependency, and closeness (Pianta 2001). Conflict, as its name implies, encompasses expressions of negative emotions and indicates that there is little rapport between educator and child. Poor academic and behavioral outcomes typically ensue from this type of relationship. A dependency relationship is one in which the child is overly dependent on the educator and feels possessive of them. It too leads to poor outcomes, including attachment disorders. Closeness is, of course, the optimal type of relationship. Here, there are positive emotions and warmth between both educator and child. It leads to the optimistic outcomes every educator strives for.

As necessary as close connections are between early childhood professionals and children, the reality of trying to form a bond with a child who is aggressive or seemingly pushing you away at every opportunity is not necessarily easy. Trauma can change the brain's architecture so that it jeopardizes a child's ability to bond with educators (Craig 2016). It takes a concerted effort on your part to get through the child's defenses, to not take challenging behaviors personally, and to reframe children's negative actions as calls for help. It is an unfortunate reality that those children who seem the least loveable are usually the ones who need your affection the most.

There are some basic things you can do to secure close relationships when they don't happen automatically. The following list contains ideas you can use to help you better forge a connection with children (Craig 2016; Jennings 2019a; Joseph & Strain 2004; Sorrels 2015; Wright 2017):

> Be genuine in your belief that connecting with children is your most important task as an educator and that social and emotional development are the key to academic and life success.

> Always keep in mind that oppositional or defiant behavior is not aimed at you personally but could have been caused by adversity that may have affected children's neural development.

> Be proactive in establishing the relationship. Don't expect it to evolve naturally on its own. The more active you are in pursuing connections, the more likely children are to respond positively.

> At the start of the year, conduct a home visit, if possible, so that children get to know you in familiar surroundings. Having already met you at home takes the pressure off the child to get to know you in the school environment. A pre-introduction also takes away the competition children often feel in getting their new teacher to notice them. (There is detailed information on making home visits in Chapter 8.)

> Monitor your own internal state as you react to children's challenging behaviors. Maintain objectivity at all times to facilitate self-regulation in children.

> Encourage children to look inside of themselves so they can see what's going on and what they are feeling: "What is your head telling you about what happened on the playground?" As children learn to observe what is happening internally, they can choose to focus on positive emotions and relationships over negative ones.

> Take an interest in children's lives outside of the program by remembering details and asking questions: "Does your cat, Cuddles, still greet you at the door when you come home from school?"

> Learn about each child's preferences, interests, background, and culture so that you can interact in ways that build on this knowledge. By having this information, your conversations with each child will be relevant and interesting to the child, respectful of the child's background and identity, and enjoyable. So if Lucas is fascinated by the dinosaur *Kamuysaurus japonicus*, figure out a way to bring the *Kamuysaurus japonicus* into your conversations, dramatic play scenarios, songs, and block constructions.

> Don't forget to share information about yourself with children so that the relationship between you is reciprocal. Let children know, for example, that you used to play drums in a garage band when you were younger. Although young children often are shocked to know that their educators have a life outside of the program, being able to see you as a person who is not focused on teaching 100 percent of the time can remove barriers.

> Greet each child by name in the morning and say goodbye to each child by name at the end of the day. Using the children's names when interacting with them lets children know that you know who they are and that they are important to you.

> Contact or send a card to children who are absent. When they return to the program, let them know how much they were missed.

> Send books or projects home in a backpack so that you keep a connection with the child during hours outside of the program.

> Praise and thank children for specific helpful and positive actions when appropriate and in front of others: "Ramon, thank you for helping Miles put away the puzzle he was playing with. There were a lot of pieces to pick up, and you were a good friend to help out." Or say, "You did a great job of paying attention today" rather than the universal "Good job." If you need to correct a child, do it in private so they do not feel ashamed or scolded in front of others: Ask Emi to go with you away from the water table where she has been playing, kneel down to her height, and quietly tell her, "Emi, I know that you enjoy playing with the scoops, but you can't be dumping the water on other children's heads. You know how that upset everyone and how we had to dry Eduardo and Luna off. How about if you take a turn using the waterwheel? I think you'll find that great fun. Let's get it off the shelf together and we can take it to the water table."

> Find something to compliment a child on in front of family members while the child is listening, at arrival or pickup. "Ms. Campbell, I'm sure that you'll enjoy reading the book on pandas with Kyleigh tonight that I put in her backpack. She's become our classroom panda expert."

> Ask children who enjoy physical touch if they would like a hug, and if they would, interact with affectionate touch—fist bumps, high fives, and gentle hugs. Bear in mind, though, that some children who have experienced trauma are touch averse, and educators do not want to trigger fearful memories by touching them—no matter how well intentioned the touch is.

> Use a soft, playful voice when talking with children. Avoid anything that sounds threatening, sarcastic, or aggressive. At the same time, don't revert to baby talk or sing-song patter. Children experiencing stress pay attention to the tone of your voice and take cues from it.

> Be mindful of your posture and facial expressions around children. These too carry messages that affect children.

> When talking to a child, look them in the eye and give them your full attention. This often means getting down to the child's height. Let children feel that there is no one more important in the world than they are every time you are together.

> Be at the children's side when they feel uncomfortable or out of place or when something triggers a survival reaction. Even if a child makes you feel unwanted and unhelpful, be there for them despite hurtful words or actions, making sure that you are not entering the child's personal body space. Your nurturing presence will make a difference.

> Let children know that your relationship can withstand strong emotions and uncomfortable feelings. By not showing surprise, discomfort, or alarm when a child becomes overly emotional, you reassure children that they are not alone.

> When things go badly, don't pretend they didn't. At departure time tell the child, "I'm sorry we had some difficult times today. Let's try to make tomorrow better!"

> Keep in mind that you are getting something out of the relationships, too. Relationships ought never be one-sided. A healed child is a happy child and is far easier to teach. This will make you feel good about your skills and proud of your abilities. At the same time, getting to know children as people most certainly will enrich your life and expand your horizons.

If you struggle to forge a caring relationship with a child, ask your supervisor or a colleague to watch your interactions with the child and offer suggestions. Remember that every relationship with every child doesn't have to be an idyllic special bond. What the relationship needs to be, though, is honest, positive, and consistent. Don't give up on a child no matter how rough the journey seems. The result promises great rewards for you both.

Help Children Form Strong Friendships with Their Peers

Trauma negatively affects a child's ability to make friends in the same way that it ravages relationships with close adults. Anger and ill temper can push other children away. A diminished ability to read faces and nonverbal cues makes many children who have experienced trauma misinterpret other children's behavior. Children with trauma backgrounds often project their own guilt, shame, and anger onto their peers and ascribe malicious or devious behavior to others when there is no such intent (Miller, n.d.; Peterson 2016).

In addition, trauma can slow children's development of the social skills needed to invite other children to play and be close to them. And for children who don't know how to share or who don't have well-developed emotional regulation, perspective-taking, and empathic abilities, friendships will rarely occur on their own (Meyers 2014).

For young children, peer friendships are nearly as important as their relationship with you. Children need at least one or two close friends to grow and develop, be healthy, and prosper (Child Mind Institute, n.d.). Researchers attribute the following benefits to preschool and kindergarten friendships (Derhally 2016; Peterson 2016):

> Better developed social and emotional skills

> Increased sense of belonging

> Decreased stress

> Better understanding of the rules of conversation

> More sensitivity to others' viewpoints

> Better understanding of how to interact with others

> Less deviant behavior

> Protection from being victimized or bullied by peers

> Increased self-esteem

> Improved school performance

All children will benefit from these advantages, but they are particularly critical for children who have experienced trauma. Improbably, even though these children are likely most in need of peer relationships, trauma has positioned them to be the least attractive to others as potential friends because they are likely to appear bossy, mean, disinterested, or stubborn.

You may need to guide and support children who have experienced trauma to make friends since the process is not likely to occur without intervention. Try some of these approaches to help children connect with their peers:

> Model being a friend and what you like about being a friend: "Ms. Winter and I are friends as well as coteachers. I know that if I ask her to take over circle time, she would do her very best not just because she is a good teacher but because she would never let me down."

> Build on a child's strengths as a way to encourage the development of skills. "Becky, I think Fatima really appreciated that you invited her to play in the dramatic play center. I bet next time she would want to stay and play longer if you asked her what role she would like to play instead of telling her she has to be the baby. Would you like to try inviting her again?"

> Work with children in reading others' facial cues. "Let's look in a mirror together. When I get mad, the muscles in my face tighten and I squeeze my lips together. What does your face look like when you are mad?"

> Help children become emotional detectives by using feeling posters. "I can tell this little girl is upset because she is frowning. How do you think this little boy who is smiling is feeling?"

> Pair up potential friends to play together: "Would you boys like to sort through the leaves we collected on our nature walk this morning? That's great that you picked an interest area where you both can have fun."

> Stay close to children to offer guidance and reassurance when they are first playing together as potential friends: "While you are riding trikes together, I'll be directing traffic like a policeman."

> Help children enter play activities if they don't yet have the skills on their own: "Brixton, shall we go over to the dramatic play center together? It looks like a bunch of children are running a restaurant. I bet they need some customers."

> When one child rejects another, sit with the rejected child and debrief the situation to see what went wrong and how the situation might have been resolved more positively: "From what I saw, Kylo wanted to join you in playing with the rain shower. When you wouldn't let him, he moved away from the water table and left you alone, which made you cry. How do you think Kylo felt when you wouldn't let him play with the rain shower? What might you have done differently if you wanted him to stay at the water table?"

> Pair children together to work on a task or project, especially picking situations where the child who has a trauma experience can be a leader: "Emilio, why don't you and Dakari work on the computer program together. Dakari, Emilio is very skilled in using this program, so he will be a big help to you."

> Take photos of children playing together and share them during group meetings. You might also post them on room dividers near where the play took place. In front of the children in the photos, show the pictures to visiting adults: "Mrs. Thompson, I want to show you a photo we took today of Tomo and Makenna peeling carrots for our snack. They worked very well together, and we all enjoyed having our carrots peeled for us."

> Read children books about friendships such as *The Adventures of Beekle: The Unimaginary Friend* (by Dan Santat). Try reading a book to pairs of would-be friends or to individual children, discussing the how-tos of making friends.

> Praise children when you see them being good friends, as positive reinforcement: "Andre, what a good friend you are to JuJu. I know how much he appreciates your helping him mop up the paint he spilled."

Helping children make friends will facilitate their recovery and enhance their school experience. This skill will enrich their lives both now and in the future.

Mindfulness as a Tool for Building Relationships and Other Needed Skills

Mindfulness involves an interface between our minds and bodies and the environment. It is the practice of becoming intensely aware of what you are sensing and feeling in the present moment, with an open, accepting, nonjudgmental mind. In child terms, mindfulness is noticing how your body feels and what you see, hear, touch, smell, and taste. It is also being aware of what your mind is doing (Bergstrom 2015). There are a variety of ways to help children practice mindfulness, including meditation, guided imagery, and breathing exercises that help relax the body and mind and reduce stress. These practices will be explored in a later section.

As simple as it sounds, mindfulness is an effective tool in dealing with the toxic stress of trauma and clearing children's minds so they can better focus and connect with others. Research has demonstrated that mindfulness is an evidence-based intervention that promotes self-regulation and resilience while mitigating the effects of ACEs and other traumas (Ortiz & Sibinga 2017).

Though mindfulness has a long history, it has become a favored tool of modern education. Because of its ability to help users steer their attention to the present moment, it can be used with young children to calm their minds, regulate their emotions, lower negative emotional reactivity, decrease depression, and better connect to their educators and peers.

In addition to a body of research documenting the ability of mindfulness to make relationships more positive and stronger in general (Greenberg 2017), there is specific research showing that mindfulness predisposes preschool teachers to having higher-quality relationships with the children they teach (Becker, Gallagher, & Whitaker 2017). It also works the other way: mindfulness is one of the most important tools in your repertoire to help children make connections with both you and their peers by helping them self-regulate and become attuned to others. When using mindfulness with children who have a history of trauma, you'll want to make certain accommodations so that the experience doesn't inadvertently trigger fears. These techniques will be explained in detail in a later section.

Why Mindfulness Works

Since the mid-1970s, mindfulness has shifted in US culture from being regarded solely as a religious practice to including secular practices for reducing stress and addressing medical needs and also as a way to accomplish goals and make users feel more grateful and happy. While trauma causes negative changes to the brain's architecture (see Chapter 3), mindfulness can counteract some of these outcomes by making positive structural and functional changes to the traumatized brain (Manitoba Trauma Information & Education Centre, n.d. a). These changes enable individuals who have experienced trauma and who practice mindfulness to pause before reacting and choose a better course of action, even under stress (Manitoba Trauma Information & Education Centre, n.d. b).

Mindfulness has made its way into many early childhood curricula because it is particularly well suited to young children, taking advantage of what is happening in their developing brains (Semple et al. 2010). Neuroscientists have found that mindfulness has a significant impact on a young child's amygdala, the part of the brain that helps process emotion (Gaffrey et al. 2013). MRI brain scans of preschoolers and kindergarten-age children reveal that when children experience negative emotions such as those related to trauma, the activity in the amygdala increases substantially. For children this age who are also depressed, the amygdala activity has been described as going into "overdrive."

Mindfulness activities enable the amygdala to more effectively process children's fearful and anxious thoughts, thus counteracting some of the negative outcomes of trauma. The brain changes that result from practicing mindfulness lead to greater emotional regulation and an increasing ability to tolerate the vicissitudes of life and the peaks and valleys of relationships (Manitoba Trauma Information & Education Centre, n.d. a). Because mindfulness strengthens parts of the brain associated with the development of empathy, it has been shown to help children who practice it become more skilled at reading others' emotional cues, a social skill that is helpful in making friends and connecting with others (Tang, Hölzel, & Posner 2015).

In addition to improving children's physical, social, and emotional well-being,

> Mindfulness can *contribute directly to the development of cognitive and performance skills and executive function.* It can help young people pay greater attention, be more focused, think in more innovative ways, use existing knowledge more effectively, improve working memory, and enhance planning, problem solving, and reasoning skills. (Weare 2012, 2)

How to Incorporate Mindfulness into Your Program

This section will look at general techniques for using mindfulness with a group. In the next section, we will give you specific techniques to use with children who need mindfulness customized for them because of their trauma backgrounds.

To be most effective, mindfulness should be an integral part of the curriculum—an ongoing daily event, not something that's used when a problem appears. Many teachers find that doing mindfulness exercises at the start of the day helps children ease their anxiety and sets the tone for having a good day.

You'll want to plan how to introduce mindfulness activities to your group instead of trying to jump right in, as some children—particularly those with a trauma history—may not be emotionally regulated enough to focus on the mindfulness process. A good way to begin is by doing an emotional release activity with the whole group. One possible exercise is to have all the children bend their arms at their elbows and close their hands into fists. Then have everyone squeeze their fists as hard as they can to get all of the energy out of their bodies. In this tension-free state, they will be more receptive to the power of mindfulness. You can do this activity anytime, whether with a large or small group or an individual child.

Most mindfulness activities center on doing deep breathing exercises and becoming aware of one's surroundings and actions. In general, unless a child with a history of trauma is uncomfortable focusing on their body and breathing deeply, you can use breathing as your introduction to mindfulness. Breath is considered an anchor to focusing on the present moment. By becoming aware of your breath as you inhale and exhale, your mind becomes focused on the act of breathing, and you become calm, as it is difficult to focus simultaneously on distracting thoughts and the act of breathing.

You can do the following breathing activity together with the whole group or with individual children or small groups:

1. Locate a comfortable place such as the calming center that is removed from commotion.

2. Sit in a chair with your feet flat on the floor. Sit up straight. Place your hands in your lap. Relax your facial muscles. Close your eyes to help you focus, if it does not upset you to do so. Adjust your body so that you are totally comfortable.

3. Take an exaggerated breath, inhaling deeply through your nose (count to 4), hold your breath (count to 2), and exhale slowly through your mouth (count to 4). Continue breathing this way.

4. As you breathe, notice where you feel your breath in your body. Is it in your stomach? Your chest? Your throat?

5. As you continue breathing, you'll probably find your mind wandering. This is perfectly normal and nothing to fret about. Just bring your thoughts back to your breathing and how it feels in your body.

6. Keep breathing like this for five minutes, or as long as you can. If you lose focus, gently bring your thoughts back. Keep your body relaxed.

7. When you are done, congratulate yourself on taking the time to do mindful breathing. Repeat this exercise daily or anytime you feel stressed.

To introduce this activity, you might choose to show children a cartoon video from *PBS Parents* featuring a song with Daniel Tiger, "When You Feel So Mad You Want to Roar," about the importance of mindful breathing (use the internet search words "daniel tiger deep breath" to find a link to the video). Afterward, lead the children in singing along with the refrain: "When you feel so mad that you want to roar, take a deep breath and count to four."

Here are some additional resources on exercises to do during your mindfulness sessions:

> *Planting Seeds: Practicing Mindfulness with Children*, by Thich Nhat Hanh

> *Sitting Still Like a Frog: Mindfulness Exercises for Kids*, by Eline Snel

> *Meditation Is an Open Sky: Mindfulness for Kids*, by Whitney Stewart

Special Considerations in Using Mindfulness with Children Who Have a Trauma History

One important point about doing mindfulness exercises with children who have experienced trauma is that mindfulness is not a one-size-fits-all exercise. You need to individualize your approach to meet children's situations. The same principles that guide TIC (see Chapter 9 for a fuller discussion) can be applied to mindfulness. In fact, some practitioners suggest calling this approach *trauma-informed mindfulness* (Himelstein, n.d.).

The reason you need to wear a trauma lens when doing mindfulness is that some children (and adults) who have been exposed to trauma may become triggered by traditional methods if you blindly apply them to everyone. In these instances, rather than reaping the powerful benefits of mindfulness, these children will become retraumatized. To illustrate, many mindfulness activities, such as the one above, suggest that participants close their eyes to better focus on themselves. For some participants, though, closing their eyes can trigger fears related to the trauma. Clinical psychologist Sam Himelstein notes, "You never want to force people to close their eyes. That alone can cause trauma for some kids. The goal is not to turn people into meditation monks. It's just about learning to turn inwards and practice self-awareness" (Schwartz 2019).

So, suggest to children that they can either close their eyes or leave them open—whichever they are more comfortable doing. If you find that children want to keep their eyes open, you might ask them to look at a spot in front of them rather than at anyone in the group so that no one feels that others are staring at them.

Rather than focus on their breath, some children might do better concentrating on the sensations of their hands resting on their thighs, their feet touching the ground, or the feeling of their bottoms on a cushion (Treleaven 2019). Other experts suggest that for some children, it's better to take the focus off their bodies altogether and have them listen to noises in the room or outdoors (Dorado & Zakrzewski 2013). Some children will benefit from adding movement to meditation exercises (Treleaven 2019). Try encouraging children to walk or stretch to help them stay present if needed.

Finally, start slowly and work on exercises in small intervals to ensure that children become comfortable with the process. Familiarize yourself with all of the exercises you will be doing ahead of time so that you can be fully attuned to the children's needs and not focusing on trying to figure out what has to be done at the same time you are introducing the activities.

The key to successfully using mindfulness with children who have experienced trauma is to form nurturing relationships with children (Schwartz 2019). When children trust you, they will let you help them. Together, you can customize mindfulness activities so that every child has access to this powerful tool for removing anxiety, fostering happiness, and connecting with others.

Forest Bathing

A variation of mindfulness that is gaining in popularity with participants of all ages, especially those who have experienced trauma, is forest bathing, or *shinrin-yoku*, as it is called in Japanese. It refers to taking in the atmosphere of the forest in a mindful way.

The idea of forest bathing has existed for a long time. However, it wasn't until 1982 that forest bathing was looked to as a wellness strategy by medical professionals in Japan. Researchers, primarily in Japan and South Korea, have amassed a strong body of scientific literature on the medicinal benefits of spending time with trees. They have found that forest bathing is a mindful way of reducing stress and boosting immunity and mood. It also improves children's attention, focus, and memory (Biemans 2018).

There are two underlying reasons why mindfully being in the forest benefits people. First, there is a higher concentration of oxygen in the forest than in urban settings. Second, trees release compounds known as phytoncides. These natural oils are known to reduce stress and lower both blood pressure and heart rate when inhaled. As we breathe in the scent of the forest, we take in compounds that relax us and benefit our health.

In addition to forest bathing's documented health benefits, the following social and emotional benefits are particularly important for children who have experienced trauma (Nature at the Confluence, n.d.):

> Deeper friendships and relationships

> Increased sense of happiness

> Clearer intuition

> Increased flow of energy

> Increased capacity to communicate with nature

One final and important word about forest bathing—despite its name, it doesn't have to take place in a forest. It can involve a visit to a park or a nature walk outside your school or program. The only necessity is that there be a connection with nature. Communion with grass, shrubs, plants, flowers, birds, squirrels, butterflies, and worms as well as trees provides the benefits of *shinrin-yoku*.

Whether conducted in the great outdoors or indoors in your program, practicing mindfulness can be an incredible tool for facilitating children's emotional regulation, focus, empathy, and connection to others. You can look to mindfulness to both help children heal and solidify your relationship with the children you teach.

Tips for Interacting with Children

Once you have established a working relationship with children, one of the best ways to maintain it and see it grow further is through positive interactions. Here are some suggestions on communicating with children to facilitate your ongoing connection.

Follow the child's lead. Take cues from the child as to how much information they can comprehend and process. Listen to what children ask, and answer only the question being asked. Then, wait for the next question. Many adults tend to give more information than the child is looking for.

With preschoolers and kindergarteners, you can ask them, "What is your head telling you about . . . ?" This will let you see what information they have, work to correct misconceptions, and let them know you are there for them.

When talking to children about traumatic events in the news, encourage their questions and let them know you will answer them honestly and to the best of your ability. There is no specific way to phrase the information; it will depend on the situation. You can keep it simple: "In [city], which is close to [far from] here, some people got hurt. Many people are working to try to make sure this doesn't happen again. It is okay if thinking about it is scary or bothers you. We are here to take care of each other."

You can also turn to children to ask how you might help them: "I notice that you seem sad today and don't want to play with any of your friends. Is there something that I can do to help you feel better?" If the child doesn't know or looks at you blankly, then make a suggestion: "Would you like to come with me to the calming center and blow some bubbles together?"

Make sure you adjust your interactions not just for the children's ages but also for the presence of any developmental delays or other factors that would affect how children comprehend the information. Questions may persist and come out of nowhere, so be available for the children.

Answer the true question being asked.
At their core, children who have a trauma history are wondering "Am I safe?" In answering children's questions, don't make any empty promises. Avoid saying something like "There won't be any more fires. I promise." Because there might be. You can better serve children by reminding them of the people in their lives who are working to keep them safe—first responders, teachers, families, and even friends. You can also remind children of the many ways you keep them safe every day, such as holding their hands to cross the street.

If appropriate, also remind children of the plans that are in place to protect them. Talk about the purpose of fire drills and sheltering in place. This can be as simple as saying, "We practice fire drills so if there ever is a problem, we will know what to do and be able to do it right away!" Or "We practice sheltering in place so if something or someone is in the school who shouldn't be there, we know what to do to stay safe." You can tell them about all the people who will step in to take care of them and protect them if necessary.

Help children process your responses.
From infancy, children are tuned in to the reaction of trusted adults around them. How you respond to events, or even to children's questions, gives them a sense of how worried they should be. While it is okay to have upsetting feelings and even to show those feelings, you also need to model how to cope with them in productive ways.

As children think about and process the information, watch for changes in their behavior. They may be anxious or fearful for their safety or the safety of their loved ones. They may complain of headaches or stomachaches, or you might see changes in how they eat, sleep, and concentrate. Children may withdraw or act out, and even older children may be clingy and in need of more interaction. You will have to trust your knowledge of each child to know when these are normal parts of reacting to the information and when you need to suggest that families contact a medical or mental health professional.

Seeing how children process and cope with difficult situations will help you figure out how much to discuss and in what ways and what contexts. Also remember that young children deal with events differently than adults. They may ask a few questions, then seem to forget about it, only to have it pop up much later. Let them go at their own pace.

Be nurturing, affectionate, and sensitive. Children need to know you care—even when they might seem like they are pushing you away. They need to know that they are valued and important to you. You can reassure most children with a hand across the back or a hug. However, as mentioned in earlier in this chapter, some children are touch averse, especially if there's been sexual or physical abuse in their past. Their behavior may look like rejection, but it rarely is. Indeed, it almost never has anything to do with you, so you should not take it personally if a child doesn't want any physical contact with you. It's their survival mechanism telling them they should be wary.

Even when children enjoy physical closeness, experts recommend that you not interrupt a child at play or engaged in an activity to hug them. Traumatized children often have attachment issues, and an unexpected overture of affection can be alarming. Even more triggering is telling a child "Give me a hug." While your intent is to have a tender moment, children who have experienced trauma tend to interpret such comments as commands. And commands, which are signs of power, once again link power with physical intimacy in the child's mind.

For children who find closeness off-putting, find other ways to show you care. Smile, talk in a warm voice, and show a kind demeanor to let a child who is frightened by intimacy know you care.

Remember that traumatized children are part of a learning community. Every child in your class has a need for and a right to your best efforts as a teacher. If everyone in the program is affected by a trauma, such as a nature-related disaster (e.g., tornado, flood, hurricane, wildfire, earthquake), you will obviously want to discuss and address the trauma with the entire class. Certainly, children will react differently to the event and require individualized responses, but this type of event requires the whole class's attention.

During the morning meeting or with table group discussions during lunch, carve out time to talk about the disaster with the children. Children are bound to have misconceptions. They hear adults talking, overhear the news on TV, and have difficulty making cause-and-effect associations with what they've observed. Offer reassurances based on facts, and be there with plenty of support.

To help children further process the experience, read books to the group such as *Elmer and the Flood* by David McKee or *Tornadoes!* by Gail Gibbons, choosing whichever books match the trauma-inducing events. The commonly shared event can also be addressed through dramatic play or puppet shows. Because it is a common experience, all the children will have something to add to the play scenarios and can offer support and empathy to one another.

Likewise, secondhand experiences that affect the community are shared by the entire group. For example, a shooting at a nearby high school will permeate the lives of all who live in the area. Some of the children might even have family members, neighbors, or babysitters who were involved in the incident firsthand. You'll want to talk about the experience with the group much as you would do if children experienced the trauma themselves.

When dealing with ACEs, however, the situation is quite different. You don't have a whole group with a shared experience. You have individual children in your program who have individual exposures to different types of trauma, and you probably have some, if not many, children who have not experienced any trauma. Because you do not want to single out the children who have experienced trauma and make them feel different, have one-on-one conversations with these children. Protect trauma-exposed children from other children's curiosity, and do not allow other children to interfere with the healing process. Classmates do not need to know about the intimate trauma their peers are dealing with. You want to respect the traumatized child's and family's privacy.

At the same time, bear in mind that all the children in your class are your responsibility—not just those who are hurting from trauma. In addition, it is not good educational practice to burden children with stories of trauma. Knowing about what has happened to their friends and classmates can be very scary and stir children's own fears and anxieties.

It is natural and exemplary to want to give the children who have experienced trauma all the support and guidance you can. Your heart will naturally go out to them, as well it should. But you don't want to give them everything that's in you at the expense of the rest of the group.

Be the supportive educator a child needs and deserves to heal and thrive, but remember you have a whole community of learners to teach and support. Moreover, as already noted, there will likely be children in your program who have experienced trauma you don't know about. They have the same need for a close relationship with you as the children whose trauma backgrounds you know about.

A Path Forward

By being the caring, trusted educator children need, you can form that bond that experts and researchers have declared so important to children's recovery and success. Having a close relationship with the children you teach is something most teachers naturally want to do but cannot always make happen. We hope the strategies and tips in this chapter will enable you to do this with all the children you work with, including the most resistant children frightened by trauma.

In Chapter 7, you will see how the bond you have forged with children can be used to help children heal and learn through play.

CHAPTER
Seven | The Healing Power of Play

The importance of play in children's resilience, functioning, and learning is well documented (Yogman et al. 2018). Play optimizes development and helps children manage toxic stress. Through their interactions with materials and playmates (whether other children or adults), children practice and hone needed skills such as planning, collaborating, negotiating conflicts, and taking on new roles. Play builds a prosocial brain that can engage and interact with others in nurturing, empathic ways. At the same time, it is a medium for gaining school readiness skills such as executive function, language, and math reasoning. Play is vital to children's mastery of gross and fine motor skills, coordination, balance, and other physical development milestones. As they accomplish all these things, children develop confidence and competence.

It is not an exaggeration to say that nearly every learning goal you set for children can be mastered through play. It even helps children become better people and citizens, supporting their developing skills at following directions, compromising, persevering, and taking pride in their accomplishments.

Benefits of Play When There Is Trauma

Play also has a crucial role in helping children heal from trauma. Play and stress are closely linked (Yogman et al. 2018). As the amount of play increases, levels of the stress hormone cortisol go down. Play also activates norepinephrine, which increases the brain's plasticity. According to Yogman and colleagues (2018), "Play, especially when accompanied by nurturing caregiving, may indirectly affect human brain functioning by modulating or buffering adversity and by reducing toxic stress to levels that are more compatible with coping and resilience."

Sorrels (2015, 203–4) cites several benefits of play that are particularly important for children who have faced trauma: play facilitates brain organization and healthy development, disarms fears, mimics important and purposeful behavior, allows children to regain their voice, reduces shame and helps children regain a sense of competence, and gives children an avenue for self-expression. Let's look more closely at these benefits:

1. **Play facilitates brain organization and healthy development.** During play, brain cells organize and move to various regions of the brain, creating critical brain architecture. Specifically, play makes the prefrontal cortex—the brain's executive center for regulating emotions, planning, and solving problems—grow and work faster.

2. **Play disarms fears.** Because children are free to choose where and with whom to play; what toys, material, and equipment they want to use; and how long they want to play, they have control over the activity. This leads to a sense of security.

3. **Play mimics important and purposeful behavior.** By trying out dramatic play scenarios such as having a family dinner or being a doctor, teacher, astronaut, or hairdresser, children learn needed life skills like planning, organizing, scheduling, negotiating conflicts, and celebrating successes.

4. **Play allows children to regain their voice.** During play children can express their fears, hopes, dreams, and needs in a safe place where they won't be chided, ridiculed, or bullied. Play validates children and enables them to be their authentic selves, even when they do this by becoming imaginary others.

5. **Play reduces shame and helps children regain a sense of competence.** Many children with a background of abuse, violence, or neglect grow up thinking their needs don't matter. They may see their circumstances as being their fault. Low self-esteem and shame often take root. Through play, children can make inroads against these defeatist feelings as they solve problems and learn new skills. A sense of competence, pride, and confidence may be feelings they have never experienced before or that are just now being restored.

6. **Play gives children an avenue for self-expression.** A child who is feeling fearful might choose dark colors to paint with, pound on clay, soothe themselves in water play, move like a snake to music, play a loud drum, or cover themselves in a parachute outdoors. On a more joyous day, a child might build a rocket ship from blocks, jump wildly to music, make a mobile that dances in the wind, or put on a skit about an optimistic gopher.

A Right to Play?

The United Nations Convention on the Rights of the Child (UN OHCHR 1989) has long established play as a universal right for every child: "Parties recognize the right of the child to rest and leisure, to engage in play and recreational activities appropriate to the age of the child and to participate freely in cultural life and the arts."

Two primary factors, however, have kept this promise of a right to play from being a reality for many young children. One reason is a widespread educational belief that play is frivolous and children in early education programs should concentrate on academic pursuits in contexts that are free of play. This idea flourishes despite evidence that play is the best context for learning for young children.

This unfounded push to impose an academic philosophy at the expense of play has created inequities that are reinforced by the second factor: stereotypes and racism. The push to impose an academic philosophy is often done with the intent of helping children of color and children in low-income communities improve academically. There is a false belief that scripted curriculum, worksheets, coloring books, flashcards, and the like will provide children with the skills they need to prosper academically (Kuschner 2012).

> Looking at the ever-present push for traditional academics, and the longstanding narrative regarding underserved students who need to be "readied for kindergarten," play is now actively marginalized by an educational system that denies equal access and opportunity to play—all too often falling along racially segregated lines, as well as the class and language statuses of the children they serve. Herein lies the crux of one of the most critical equity issues in our field of education today: defining and deciding who has the right to play. (Beloglovsky & Grant-Groves 2019, 57)

This situation most negatively affects Black boys, who are frequently labeled "problem children" who misuse play and could make better use of their time by paying attention to academics (Ladson-Billings 2011). For many, play becomes an infrequent privilege at best.

Despite pressures to limit play, play is a pinnacle of early childhood education theory and practice that has been validated by biology and research (Hirsh-Pasek et al. 2009; Mardell et al. 2016; Milteer & Ginsburg 2011; Singer, Golinkoff, & Hirsh-Pasek 2006; Whitebread et al. 2009; Yogman et al. 2018; Zigler, Singer, & Bishop-Josef 2004; Zosh et al. 2017). It is up to early childhood educators to make play *every* child's right.

The Impact of Trauma on Play

Trauma can affect how and what children play. Consider the following examples:

> Everyday events may trigger a child's reaction and can cause children to become scared or aggressive or to shut down: While watching Sebine "cook" breakfast in the home center of the dramatic play area, Maurice thinks about all the times he has been hungry at home and didn't have anything for breakfast, and he suddenly gets angry. He goes over to the table where other children are seated and pushes all the tableware off the table, to everyone's surprise and shock.

> Children may re-enact trauma they have experienced, witnessed, or heard about secondhand: Following an outbreak of a virus that closed schools in their community, Emilio and Jayden spend much of their play time in the dramatic play area pretending to be doctors taking care of sick people.

> Following trauma, children's ability to connect socially with others may be inhibited: During outdoor choice time, Saroj stands alone on the playground watching the other children play. When his teacher comes over to encourage him to join one of the other children, he buries his face in her side.

> Children with a trauma history often have difficulty navigating conflicts with peers: Marcius places people figures in a LEGO bus and drives it over a "highway." Dion, who was emotionally abused in the past, announces that he wants the people figures. Marcius tells him he's using them now, but when the bus comes back, Dion can play with them. Dion snaps back, "I want them now." He then grabs the bus and shakes the people out, leaving an unhappy Marcius in tears.

> Children affected by trauma may be unable to concentrate, focus, and complete tasks: While working on a puzzle, Mattie picks up a puzzle piece and puts it down. She repeats this pattern with three other pieces, not trying to fit any pieces into the frame but preferring to look around the room.

> Children may have difficulty processing what happened during trauma and revisit it in play: "I took the baby doll to the hospital, but she died anyway. She was bad and got punished. That's what happened to my mama."

> A child's reaction to trauma may include extreme concern for others' safety and well-being: Lilly stores all of the puppets under the puppet stage, refusing to let anyone else play with them or move them elsewhere. "They have to hide so no one will be able to hurt them."

Using Play to Address Trauma's Negative Effects

Play is not just a vehicle for observing the effects of trauma; it is more importantly a tool for stemming those effects. You can skillfully use play to promote healing, enabling children to engage in play as intended, with pleasure and joy.

Types of Play That Promote Healing

There are two types of play associated with healing: free play and guided play. Together, they are known as *playful learning* and are "pedagogical tools through which children can learn in joyful and conceptually rich ways" (Hassinger-Das, Hirsh-Pasek, & Golinkoff 2017). Playful learning is defined by three characteristics: choice, wonder, and delight (Mardell et al. 2016). It typically involves social interaction with educators or other children.

Free Play

This type of play comes to mind when you think of child-initiated play or choice time. The child is in charge of what, with whom, in what center, and for how long they play. Sorrels (2015, 202–3) describes three characteristics of free play that define it:

1. It is chosen by the child, based on individual preferences and abilities. This means that Elena may spend a significant part of the day listening to audiobooks in the library area before deciding to join two other children in making a volcano with a parent volunteer in the science center.

2. The child is motivated by the pleasure of the activity. If Pedro enjoys painting a section of a mural outdoors, he can happily spend the entire choice time engaged in this activity.

3. Children make the rules of play. So if Sophie is playing the mother in the housekeeping area and she tells Aiden, who is pretending to be her son, that it's time to stop playing video games and go to bed, Aiden can either go along with Sophie's rules or not.

Researchers have found that free play especially helps children with a trauma background gain these capabilities necessary to aid in their recovery (Mardell et al. 2016; NPR 2015):

> Sense of trust

> Emotional regulation

> Ability to make choices about their life

> Empathy

> Diminished tendencies toward violence

Guided Play

Guided play is a way teachers structure free play to achieve learning goals. For example, if you see 4-year-old Shaniqua building towers of blocks that keep falling over, you might sit down with her in the block center and ask her why she thinks her tower is falling, drawing attention to the smaller blocks being placed on the bottom. Through your questioning, you could lead Shaniqua to try placing the larger blocks on the floor with the shorter blocks atop them.

Alternatively, if Shaniqua is developmentally behind expectations for her age, to scaffold her learning you might ask her how she could support the tilting blocks, leading her to use a cushion to keep the block tower standing. Your thoughtful questioning and probing will enable children to experience a higher level of success during play, even if they are developmentally behind their peers, as happens with many children affected by trauma. Following this intervention, Shaniqua can return to her free play with the blocks. In the meantime, she will have gained new skill and have experienced success.

Guided play is the type of instruction many educators who value play are familiar with and do daily. It allows you to let children have choice in their play while you monitor their progress toward your curriculum's learning goals. Guided play is not telling the children how or what to play, but rather acting as a coach during their exploration.

"Supporting Children's Explorations in Learning Centers," on pages 65–68, shows ideas for supporting free and guided play in learning centers.

Supporting Children's Explorations in Learning Centers

Learning Center	Actions and Questions to Support the Play of Children with a Trauma History in the Center
Dramatic play	To engage in free play, children must feel safe, which means you must be aware of setups that might prove triggering. A housekeeping area can cause fear in children who associate their home with bad things happening. For support, educators can empower children playing there to control the specifics of who is in the play scenario (mother and child but not the father, for example) and what the storyline should be. The same goes for other potentially scary setups, such as a doctor's office or even a school. Help children use play scenarios to work through their fears or sadness. Some questions you might ask to guide play are ■ Who is here to help you? ■ What might make things better? ■ What would you like to tell _____? ■ What would you like to happen next?
Blocks	The block area is an ideal venue for re-creating traumas children have seen or experienced. For example, an incident involving a plane that crashed into a home in their city can be processed when a child builds a house out of blocks and then "flies" a large block into it, crashing the structure over and over again. To help a child process such an event, you might pose such questions as ■ What were you thinking in your head when the plane crashed into the house? ■ What can you do to make the people in the house safe? ■ What can you do to help the pilot? ■ What could we do to prevent another accident like this?
Math and manipulatives	Open-ended toys like LEGO bricks and magnetic blocks or letters, and collectibles such as buttons, bottle caps, keys, and nuts and bolts, offer children with trauma backgrounds the same opportunity that blocks do—the ability to impose security and order on their world. Extend children's play by asking such questions as ■ How are these bottle caps alike and different? ■ How do you know where the puzzle pieces with a straight edge should go? ■ What happens when you put a small ring on the sorter pole first? ■ How did you feel when you completed the puzzle?

(continues)

Learning Center	Actions and Questions to Support the Play of Children with a Trauma History in the Center
Library	Bibliotherapy, as described in Chapter 5, is a prime method for helping children exposed to trauma deal with their feelings and heal. Appendix 2 contains book suggestions that can be used to teach effective coping strategies. In addition to using the library area to listen to read-alouds, children may wish to also use the area to work on the computer, write, listen to recorded stories, or publish their own books. To guide them in this latter activity, you might ask such questions as ■ What do you think _____ is thinking in their head? ■ Who is there to help _____? ■ What could _____ do to make things better? ■ How can you end the story so _____ feels happy and gets what they want?
Discovery	Caring for plants and classroom pets is especially valuable for children who have experienced trauma. These activities offer a child a chance to safely develop nurturing feelings that are helpful in forging a relationship with educators and peers. Educators can expand on children's burgeoning feelings of attachment by asking such questions as ■ How do you feel after you feed the fish? ■ Do you think the fish know who you are? ■ What can our class do to make sure the plants and fish do well? ■ How does it feel to be responsible for the plants' and fishes' health and well-being?
Music and movement	Music can help children who have experienced trauma self-regulate, improve verbal language and math abilities, concentrate better, and reduce behavior problems (Foran 2009). Group singing increases endorphins and oxytocin in the brain, which relieve stress and anxiety (Sorrels 2015). Singing, dancing, and moving to music promote a sense of belonging that many children with trauma histories yearn for. Because of its many therapeutic values, educators are urged to use music beyond the confines of the music and movement center and have children ■ Sing or do movement activities during the morning and closing meetings ■ Sing or do movement activities during transitions ■ Sing along to cleanup and handwashing songs ■ Listen to soft classical music during nap or rest time

Learning Center	Actions and Questions to Support the Play of Children with a Trauma History in the Center
Art	Use the visual arts to help children give voice to feelings they can't put into words. A child might paint a black sky as a way of letting you know they have dark feelings inside them. Similarly, a figure with an upside-down smile will alert you to potentially unhappy feelings. To further find out what is going on, it helps to say, "Tell me about your painting (drawing, collage, sculpture, mobile, mural, decoration)." Some helpful questions to ask children are ■ I see your whole painting is done with orange paint. What were you thinking in your head when you chose that color? ■ You just told me this is a painting of your family. I see your mommy and daddy and baby sister. But where are you? ■ I see that the little boy has tears on his face in this painting. I wonder why. ■ How did pounding the clay make you feel?
Sand and water	The sand and water center is an ideal place for children to work through emotions. Running sand through a sieve or using an eggbeater to stir water offers children a soothing, calming experience. An angry child or one with hurt feelings can readily work through upset feelings and self-regulate in the comfort of sand or water play. To assist children, try asking questions like these: ■ What happens to the sand when it gets wet? How does wet sand feel different from dry sand? ■ How do you feel when you wash the baby doll in the water? How do you think the baby doll feels? ■ I know you are upset because Freddy said something mean to you. If you would like to punch the sand, it might make you feel less angry, and it could be fun, too. ■ How does the water feel on your skin when it falls out of the sieve?
Cooking	For many children who have experienced neglect or emotional abuse or who live in poverty, food is a triggering issue. Malnutrition is an adverse effect for some children affected by trauma. For others, food may have been used to manipulate children to do what the abuser wanted or as a show of power. As noted in Chapter 5, educators can help reverse these ill effects by having self-serve snacks available to allow children to control when and how much they eat. Encourage children by asking questions like the following: ■ How does it feel to make your own snack? ■ Which foods make you feel happiest? Why is that? ■ What part do you like best about making your own snack? ■ Why do you think it's good to wait until you are hungry to eat?

(continues)

Learning Center	Actions and Questions to Support the Play of Children with a Trauma History in the Center
Outdoors	The outdoor area offers children an opportunity to work through stress and unwanted feelings by doing gross-motor activities like climbing, swinging, throwing and running after balls, and riding. Educators can enhance the experience by asking questions or making comments like these: ■ I know you are upset right now. Try throwing the beanbag into the hoop. I think it will help you feel better. ■ What does it feel like when you jump in the pile of leaves? ■ How do you feel inside your head when you make the swing go high in the air? ■ Do you prefer to go fast or slow down the slide? Why is that?

Using Playful Learning with Children Who Are Distressed

It can be disconcerting for an adult to watch a child play "dead dog" after the child's pet dies, but it is their way of working through their ideas and emotions. You can use this as an opportunity to watch what they are doing and to clear up any misconceptions they may bring up as they play.

You don't need to intervene if the play seems to be helping them. However, if they are getting more upset or scared, consider what support you might offer, starting with the least interruptive. As a first step, don't stop the play. Instead, see if you can redirect it. If that doesn't work, you'll need to change the setting. Say, "Wow, this seems to really be upsetting the mommy doll. Let's go for a walk or sit in the library and talk about it." This lets them know that what they are feeling is okay and that you are there to help them deal with it.

Children may also draw or dictate a story to you about how they are feeling. Open-ended inquiries like "Tell me what's happening in your picture" will let them express themselves. If the trauma is not reflected in their art, that doesn't mean they don't have feelings about it. It may just mean they are not ready to delve in and deal with it at the moment or that they are expressing their feelings in a different way than you expected.

If the intensity of the play continues, if a child becomes fixated on events during play, or if you have any other causes for concern, talk with the child's family and contact a professional for guidance.

Differences Between Playful Learning and Play Therapy

Some children exposed to trauma may not know how to play in a productive way. They may lack the skills to interact with other children or not know how to take out and put away materials on their own. You may observe them hitting others, taking over dramatic play, making demands, not understanding rules, barking orders, or refusing to clean up. For these children, you will need to model how to use materials and interact with others. They may need your help to learn how to play appropriately and meaningfully so that play becomes an enjoyable learning tool for everyone.

Other children may become obsessed with re-creating the experienced trauma. They need your help to work through their fears and emerge with a better perspective. With patience and scaffolding and modeling, you can help most children play more productively and joyfully.

Sometimes, though, teachers cannot break through the wall that keeps a child from playing appropriately. The child's challenging behaviors or fears will not abate, especially if they have PTSD.

At these times, it's best to meet with the child's family and perhaps suggest that the child see a specialist known as a play therapist.

Play therapists are specialized child therapists who can help children with trauma histories by working with them to address cognitive, behavioral, and emotional challenges. These licensed mental health professionals have had specialized training to help children living with trauma or PTSD and those who have issues caused by bullying, grief and loss, abandonment, and physical and sexual abuse.

You may find it helpful to have an introductory session with a play therapist or other specialist to determine whether formal therapy is warranted. Play therapy has been proven to have successful outcomes, including improved prosocial behaviors and decreased symptomatic behaviors (Gaskill & Perry 2014). To learn more about what play therapists do and how they might help, check out the Association for Play Therapy's website (www.a4pt.org).

When Violence Is a Part of Play

A concern for many educators is how to handle children's play with violent themes, whether with toy or imaginary guns, as superheroes, or as cops and robbers. This type of play is common among all children, but for children who have experienced trauma, it may be one more way they play out their reactions and emotions and process what happened. For example, you may find a child who experienced a drive-by shooting building a tall wall of blocks in the block center and then hiding behind it, talking about how well protected they would be. This gives the child a sense of control and helps them put things in perspective.

Even if children haven't been directly exposed to a traumatic event, many have heard about them from adults or older children, seen images in the media, or live in a community that has experienced violence. All of this can work its way into their play as they try to make sense of their world. The consensus among child development experts is that children benefit from play that allows them to feel powerful—even when it involves guns and violence (Pevzner 2014). They use this play to figure out how to manage aggressive impulses while getting the chance to feel powerful in a world where they don't have much control.

If you have ever attempted to ban gun-related and violent play from your program, you likely discovered that children found a way to take their play underground or away from adult supervision. "All you are doing is telling them that their fantasies and imaginations are bad," says Jane Katch, author of *Under Deadman's Skin: Discovering the Meaning of Children's Violent Play*. "It only invites [children] to be sneaky and hide their real feelings" (Pevzner 2014).

Instead of a zero-tolerance ban, find a way to monitor and observe the play, using it as a way to discuss gun safety and thoughts and feelings about power and violence. Use children's gun and war play to help children understand how this type of play can affect other people. Pointing out when friends seem scared or anxious and helping them read the verbal and nonverbal cues for when the play should stop or move to a new location is a critical social and emotional skill many children exposed to trauma lack. It reinforces for all children that they have a right to their feelings and how they want to play and interact.

At the same time, you must be aware of boundaries and what to do if they are crossed. As with all play, if it seems to be causing anxiety or fear to the children playing it, or if they are deliberately trying to intimidate others—even after being asked repeatedly to stop—it is important to step in to redirect the play. Your knowledge of the children and what they are going through in other areas of their lives will help guide your response. If you are concerned, contact a professional to help you support the children involved.

Gun and war play usually dissipate after a while (Criswell, in Gladstone 2014). While of high interest initially, it loses its draw for most children and eventually becomes indistinguishable from other forms of dramatic play.

Tips for Using Children's Play as a Healing Agent

Allow Children Enough Time to Become Fully Engaged in Their Play

As indicated in Chapter 5, children need long stretches of uninterrupted play to become fully involved in what they are doing. Children with a trauma background may need to calm down and self-regulate before they can begin playing in a way that leads to learning. Think about children involved in a dramatic play scenario. They have to decide who is available to play and what type of scenario they want to do. Will it be at school, a laundromat, or a picnic area? Then roles have to be decided upon, dress-up clothes and shoes put on, and perhaps accessories made in the art area. Much of this takes place before children even begin their scenario. For play to achieve its many goals, you need to give it the time it needs to work.

Use Play's Repetitiveness to Desensitize Children to Their Fears

One of the major benefits of dramatic play, as noted previously in this chapter, is that children can invent scenarios that allow them to act out their fears over and over again while maintaining control. Eventually, this type of play allows most children to come to terms with their feelings.

Four-year-old Damon was traumatized by the severe flooding that took place in his community following a major hurricane. At school he refused to play at the water tub and cringed when asked to wash his hands. His mother reported that Damon refused to take a bath at night.

Damon's teacher, Ms. Livingston, noticed that Damon liked to re-create play scenarios featuring flooding rivers or pools with overflowing water. She decided it would be good for Damon to throw his feelings into his play to see where the dramatic play led him. Every day for a couple of weeks, Damon played in the dramatic play area, making up scenarios featuring floods. Sometimes the waters overflowed, causing havoc in his created world. Nearby geese flew away. Houses were destroyed. Once a baby doll drowned. During his play, Ms. Livingston talked to Damon about what was happening and how he felt, but she made no effort to stop his play, even when the doll drowned.

After two weeks of flood scenarios, Damon stopped acting scared of water. He washed his hands without incident and didn't flinch when it rained. His mother shared that Damon took a bath without fighting her. Being able to re-create the flood scenes over and over desensitized Damon to his fear.

Use Play to Offer Children Joy and Hope

By definition, play involves wonder and delight (Mardell et al. 2016). While play helps heal children wounded by trauma and teaches skills to all children, educators ought never forget that play is also fun. So share a laugh with a child as a Hula-Hoop twirls off their body. Encourage children to enthusiastically sing the cleanup song at the top of their lungs. And share a child's delight and pride as you make a frame to showcase their artwork on the wall. Children, including those with trauma backgrounds, are children first. And every child needs to savor the joys of play.

A Path Forward

Play is every child's right. For children with a history of trauma, it is also a path to recovery and healing as well as learning. In the context of play, children learn to both self-regulate and acquire new skills and concepts. Using the strategies and ideas presented in this chapter, you can help children realize their full potential as they make peace with their pasts.

In Chapter 8, you will learn how many of the same principles of TIC used with children can be applied to your partnership with the children's families.

CHAPTER
Eight   Partnering with Families

When teachers have a trusting partnership with children's families, everyone is enriched. The importance of connecting with families has long been documented by research (Colker & Koralek 2018; Halgunseth et al. 2009; Henrich & Gadaire 2008; Weiss, Caspe, & Lopez 2006) and established by every major organization and agency concerned with high-quality early childhood education (including NAEYC, Head Start, federal and state departments of education, military child care/Department of Defense Education Activity, and the National Education Association). In 2016, the US Department of Health and Human Services (HHS) and the US Department of Education (ED) issued the joint "Policy Statement on Family Engagement: From The Early Years to the Early Grades." It established recommendations on integrating family engagement into early childhood systems and programs.

When true collaborations exist between early educators and families, children feel safer, more secure, and better positioned to learn. These partnerships, often categorized under the term *family engagement,* ease children's transitions between home and school. While of benefit to all, these relationships are especially important for families with children who have lived with trauma.

What Is a Family?

What constitutes a family varies significantly. Parents may be married, single, separated, or divorced. They could be gay, straight, cisgender, transgender, or nonbinary. They may include caregivers who gave birth and those who have adopted a child or are stepparents. A family may also include siblings, blended step-siblings, or other family members such as grandparents, uncles, or aunts. The federal policy statement on family engagement defines a family as "adults who interact with early childhood systems in support of their child, to include biological, adoptive, and foster parents; grandparents; legal and informal guardians; and adult siblings" (HHS & ED 2016, 1).

For children exposed to trauma that involves separation from their parents, the role of parent extends to those who care for children outside of the family. Sometimes the courts or parents themselves will request that children temporarily or permanently live with relatives or close friends of the family who serve as temporary or permanent guardians. This is known as kinship care.

Foster care is a state-funded social program that provides temporary care for children who cannot live with their own families. Foster care is not meant to be permanent, so children typically continue to visit their own families, with reunification as the goal. While the child is out of the home, public services are provided to help facilitate a healthy reunion. Nearly half of the children in foster care return to their families of origin within six months (Szilagy 2014). If reunification is not deemed advisable and no other option is available, a foster family may seek permanence through adoption or legal guardianship, or the child may be made eligible for adoption by another family (Sherer Law Offices, n.d.).

Resource parents are a hybrid of a foster parent and an adoptive parent. Instead of viewing their relationships with children as temporary, resource parents are positioned to adopt the children they foster. They can be anyone who is currently functioning as—or is in the process of becoming—a licensed kinship caregiver, foster parent, or legal guardian.

Adults who take in children as part of kinship care, foster care, or resource care all participate in the care and education of the children in their homes. Whether temporary or permanent, they too are the children's families.

In this chapter and throughout this book, when we use the words *parent* and *family,* we are referring to the many constellations that families represent. The principles of family engagement are inclusive to all these different family structures and relationships. Figure 6 offers some suggested language that helps all families feel accepted and included.

Family-Inclusive Language

Avoid	Why?	Instead
"parents" "mom" "dad" "mom and dad"	Not everyone accompanying a child is a parent. Grandparents, step-parents, and nannies may not identify as parents. Not all children have a mom and dad.	"grownup" "adult" "caregiver"
"son" "daughter"	The children in someone's care could be grandchildren, nieces, nephews, godchildren, etc. You may also not want to assume the gender of a child.	"children"
"extended family"	This term is usually meant to include grandparents, aunts, uncles, and cousins, but for folks of many cultures this isn't "extended" family. It's just family.	"family"
"family resemblance"	We're conditioned to look for similar features in family members, so you may see resemblance where there is none. Many families include step-parents, adoptive parents, or parents who conceived with donated eggs or sperm. Inversely, don't assume that a child who doesn't look like their caregiver is adopted—many multi-racial children resemble one parent more than the other.	Keep it to yourself
"members of a household"	Families don't always live together—for example, families with divorced parents or incarcerated parents.	"family members"

Figure 6. Examples of phrases that include all types of families. Adapted, by permission, from M. Middleton, "Family-Inclusive Language," www.margaretmiddleton.com/family-inclusion (2014). Copyright © 2014 by Margaret Middleton.

What Is Engagement?

Simply put, the difference between parent involvement and family engagement is the difference between "doing to" and "doing with." As one teacher succinctly puts it, "instead of using your mouth to give instructions to families, you use your ears to listen" (Ferlazzo 2012).

Family engagement is often referred to as a partnership or reciprocal relationship. The concept is well supported by the field and in particular by NAEYC. Embedded in NAEYC's position statement on DAP (2009) and in its early learning program standards (2018), family–teacher partnerships are also a part of NAEYC's professional standards and competencies for early childhood educators (2020) and its position statement on advancing equity (2019).

The joint statement between the HHS and the ED (2016) defines family engagement this way:

> Family engagement refers to the systematic inclusion of families in activities and programs that promote children's development, learning, and wellness, including in the planning, development, and evaluation of such activities, programs, and systems. For family engagement to be integrated throughout early childhood systems and programs, providers and schools must engage families as essential partners when providing services that promote children's learning and development, nurture positive relationships between families and staff, and support families. (1)

This definition can best be put into place when a program encompasses the following three principles of family engagement and 10 family engagement practices (HHS & ED 2016; Koralek, Nemeth, & Ramsey 2019; Maryland Family Engagement Coalition 2016).

Family Engagement Principles

These principles lay the groundwork for a successful partnership between families and educators.

Ensure that communication is two-way and reciprocal. In the following example, a teacher listens to a family member's idea for helping a child deal with separation anxiety.

> In meeting with 3-year-old Enoch's aunt about Enoch's struggles at drop-off time, his aunt suggested to his teacher that it might be helpful if Enoch brought his favorite stuffed animal to the program with him and wanted to know if that was okay. His teacher responded, "That's a great idea, Ms. Adebayo. That will also give him comfort if he feels distressed during the day. I'd also like to send some feeling charts home with you that will help him identify his emotions. We use them here, too, so they will be familiar to him."

Use a strengths-based approach that builds on family members' talents, skills, and interests. The teacher in this example looks for ways to incorporate a parent's strong interests and abilities.

> When meeting with 6-year-old Anita's father, Anita's teacher says, "Mr. Cardoza, thank you for helping the children plant our own vegetable garden. It was wonderful that you brought in so much STEM learning in sorting and measuring and categorizing the plants. The children have set up a schedule for watering and weeding the garden. The best part is we'll be able to grow our own veggies for snacks."

Individualize interactions with each family. In the example below, the teacher accommodates her approach to match a family's circumstances.

> Teacher to grandfather of 4-year-old Lamont: "I know you can't get texts or emails on your phone, so would it be best for us to stay in touch about Lamont by talking together on the phone? I can give you my number and the best times to reach me. If you would do the same, I think that will work out great."

Family Engagement Practices

These practices will help you build positive relationships with families and also benefit children.

Work with family members to jointly set goals and make decisions about their child. Challenges are best solved when families team with teachers. Sometimes teachers aren't aware of problems family members observe at home.

> Mother of 4-year-old Josh to his teacher: "I would like to figure out a way with you to help Josh make friends. Ever since his dad was deployed, he's been keeping too much to himself." Teacher: "We can definitely do that. I agree that that is an excellent goal for us to be working on."

Support children through transitions in their lives. Children need support from all sides when facing life's changes and challenges.

> Teacher to the parents of 4-year-old Tonio, whom they recently adopted after fostering for a year: "Congratulations to the whole Garcia family. This is a wonderful milestone in Tonio's life. I've been reading books with him at school about adoption. He especially likes *The Best Family In The World* by Susana Lopez. I like it too because it isn't about a newborn being adopted like so many of the storybooks are. The other book I like reading with him is *Siempre, Siempre Te Querré*, by Hoda Kotb, because it is in Spanish, which I think makes him feel close to you. If you'd like, I can lend you these books and give you a list of other books about adoption that you can check out of the library."

Promote family well-being. Educators should constantly look for ways to best support children and families, as the teacher in this example does.

> Teacher to foster parent of 4-year-old Andres: "Andres has been doing just great, Ms. Jennings. He has settled in well and is very curious and eager. The reading you have been doing with him at home is paying off. He's especially interested in science. We've been reading books about weather and the night sky. On another subject, I know you are working with Andres's mother to reunify their family. I was wondering if it makes sense to have her here when we next meet to talk about Andres. If you think that's a good idea, perhaps you could ask Andres's family's social worker to make the arrangements."

Facilitate positive family–child relationships. Part of teaching is helping family members be the best parents they can be. The teacher in the following example helps parents work through sibling fights.

> Teacher to the parents of 6-year-old Antoine: "How have the guidance tips we talked about been working out? Has there been less fighting between Antoine and his siblings? I think the more secure and safe he feels, the less need he has to be aggressive. Are you observing that, too? How would you describe Antoine's behavior these days?"

Provide activities that can be done at home to support program learning. Children learn best when routines and activities they do at their program are reinforced at home, as in the example below.

> Four-year-old Ebele's mother to her teacher: "Thank you for sending home information on how to make a picture daily schedule at home like you have here. It helps for Ebele to know our after-school routine. After she gets home, she can play with her toys until it's time to help set the table for dinner. After dinner, we do dishes together, and then I'll read her a story. Knowing what's next calms her down and keeps her from getting anxious."

Connect families with other families in the program for social support and networking. Teachers can build parents' confidence, skills, and enjoyment by teaming them with fellow parents who share similar concerns and interests.

> Mother of 4-year-old Levi thanks his teacher for connecting her with other parents who are working together to rid their community of gun violence, telling her, "I feel so much stronger knowing other parents who share my needs and values. I think I'm becoming a better mother by fighting for my child."

Connect families to community support organizations and staff. As illustrated below, teachers are in a position to offer much-needed services to family members by maintaining current contact information for individuals and agencies that provide services to families with young children.

> Teacher to parents of 3-year-old Donna Lynn: I understand that you had to vacate your home because of the recent wildfires. I have a list of places offering free meals, supplies, and counseling services that might be helpful during the next few months until you can get resettled at home. Let's discuss what services you need, and I'll do my best to help you find a service provider. Our whole community is in this together. This disaster has certainly brought out the best in our neighbors."

Support families as lifelong educators of their children. In the following example, a teacher helps a parent see the special role he has in his daughter's life as both a teacher and a father.

> To the father of 5-year-old Aviva, her teacher says: "You know that you are Aviva's first and best teacher, advocate, and nurturer. After Aviva goes to kindergarten, you can continue teaching her new things at home. For example, encourage her to cook with you. When you chop vegetables, she learns about size, shape, and measurement and develops muscle skills in her hands. When you make popcorn in the microwave, you can teach her about volume and how physical states change. We have several children's cookbooks you could look at and see if you'd like to borrow."

Support families in their own educational needs and aspirations. As illustrated below, teachers have a professional obligation to help families—not just their children—thrive and flourish.

> The mother of 3-year-old Grayson, with whom she was recently reunited, to his teacher: "My social worker said it would be good for me to take some parenting classes. Is that something you can help me with?" Teacher: "Of course. I think it will help strengthen your relationship with Grayson to know how you should expect him to grow and develop as he gets older. We have a consultant who teaches child development and parent education classes on Wednesday evenings and Saturday mornings. Let me go get the fliers and we can discuss this right now."

Support families as child advocates. Advocacy enriches children, families, and the entire community. In the following example, a teacher encourages a parent to consider taking on this role.

> Teacher to resource parent of 3-year-old Dallas: "Thanks to all of the work you've been doing with Dallas at home, we are seeing enormous positive changes in his behavior. Now, instead of us dealing with meltdowns and outbursts, we see him making up songs and dictating stories to us that he illustrates. I think it would be wonderful if you would share your experience and skills with others. Do you think you might be interested in doing a workshop sometime?"

Special Considerations in Working with Families of Children Who Have Experienced Trauma

It is critical for educators to partner with families of children who have experienced trauma, not just to ensure the quality of children's learning but also to enable children to heal. Recovery from trauma involves the support of both educators and family members working together.

Principles of Trauma-Informed Family Engagement

To allay family members' stress and anxiety about meeting and working with educators, educators should consider the following core values of TIC (Meeker 2015). You are likely using variations of this guidance already, as it applies to all populations.

Ensure that when families meet with you, they feel physically and emotionally safe. To do this, begin by greeting and talking with family members in a calm, warm manner. If English is not their first language, try to say at least a few welcoming phrases in their home language. Consider serving snacks and having water or other beverages available. If a parent gets upset or agitated during a meeting, carefully think about what you can say to deflect the situation. Avoid telling someone to calm down, which often has the opposite effect. Instead say something like "Perhaps we should take a five-minute break. Can I get you some water or coffee?"

Be transparent and trustworthy. Let family members know ahead of time when and why you want to meet with them. Avoid scheduling meetings at the last minute. Make sure families understand that the purpose of all meetings is to work together to help their child heal and thrive. Most meetings should be check-ins where you focus on the whole child and review the child's progress. This means looking at what is going well and then building on the child's strengths to overcome any challenges.

To further instill trust, it's vital to keep your promises. As with interactions with children, don't make a promise unless you know you can honor it. If you make a commitment in good faith and for some reason you can't keep what was promised, apologize and find a way to make the situation better. And then do it. Being able to depend on you is a starting point in forging a relationship that works.

Share decision-making responsibilities with family members. Family engagement is all about sharing power. Even though it may sometimes feel to you and the children's families that you are in charge of sharing all the information and answers, this is not appropriate. If this is the case, you'll need to reconsider your approach, because this shouldn't be true in either practice or appearance. Family engagement works only when there is true collaboration and each partner respects what the other brings to the table.

Supporting Families in Supporting Their Children

Many of the same considerations that apply to working with children who have experienced trauma also apply to working with family members. Some parents will have experienced the same trauma their children have. Traumatic events such as these could adversely affect both children and their parents: a death in the family; a family member with serious chronic illness or who has been hospitalized; one or more family members involved in a traffic collision; an incarcerated parent; a deployed parent; a family member with substance use disorder; domestic abuse; and divorce or a custody dispute.

Even when the child's traumatic experience(s) are not shared, parents may have had their own adverse childhood experiences, which are often projected onto their children. As the research confirms, both recent traumatic experiences and the lingering effects of ACEs may trigger ongoing fight-flight-freeze responses that will influence the parents' abilities to self-regulate and the way they parent their children (Meeker 2015).

What does this mean for educators trying to forge a relationship and partner with families? First, look inward and examine your own beliefs and comfort level in dealing with families whose backgrounds or experiences may be very different from your own. Preconceived beliefs should be challenged. In this regard, Zacarian and colleagues (2017a) write:

> We have to be aware of the preconceptions, stereotypes, and myths that each of us can have about the families we work with. Some of these myths include such stereotypes as the beliefs that all poor families share the same way of being and acting, are "unmotivated and have weak work ethics," are uninvolved in their children's school because they do not value education, are linguistically deficient, and "tend to abuse drugs and alcohol" (Gorski 2008). Stereotypes such as these can and do greatly affect our capacity to work successfully with families. (105)

To combat these tendencies, educators can apply the same trauma-sensitive lenses to children's family members that they use to help children heal. If a parent raises their voice and seems combative, it may be because stress hormones have kicked in and they are in a fight mode. A parent who misses meetings and doesn't show up at an agreed-upon time may be in flight mode, not rude and uncooperative. Likewise, a parent who sits silently and seemingly tunes you out may be in a freeze response and not indifferent. Even if the parents' reactions do not stem from trauma-related causes, as with children, a trauma-informed approach will benefit all.

In addition, some parents may be sensitive because of unhappy past interactions, leading them to believe that you and other authority figures are against them. Being asked to disclose personal information can feel threatening, especially if they feel ashamed or worry they're going to be criticized. Something as simple as making eye contact may be difficult or uncomfortable for some family members.

Remember that behaviors like these tend to be chronic, largely automatic responses to stressful situations. Family members of children with trauma histories have likely had at least one negative experience in their past with social services, the justice system, or other educators. And given their past experiences with institutions, they may have difficulty trusting you.

Regaining trust and easing parents' fears will take time and patience. Keep an open mind and understand that a parent's negativity is often a coping mechanism. Consider that family members who have had only negative experiences working with professionals involved in their child's care need great courage to try once again and agree to meet with you. What a breakthrough it would be to stop old patterns and form a true working relationship with families.

Adding to these trauma-related behaviors that may appear in unexpected ways, teachers need to remember that culture also influences how families will react to you both as an educator and as an individual and to the process of family engagement. Some families regard their child's educator as an expert to be treated with deference and respect, some will be wary of your intentions and may view you as an intruder in their lives, some will challenge your knowledge and ideas, some will react hesitantly or even negatively in response to some aspect of your own culture, and others will welcome your invitations to be equal partners in their children's education.

Culture also influences family members' feelings about how the program should operate and what constitutes appropriate interactions between children and educators. If you find that a family's perspective differs from yours or your program's, your professional responsibility is to keep an open mind. Resist the temptation to jump in and set the record straight. Listen to everyone's perspective and consider why they think this way. Often viewpoints are not as far apart as they seem initially. Can adjustments be made so that everyone feels heard and respected? Cross-cultural communication requires critical listening, reflection, support, and practice.

Connecting with Families to Benefit Children

Teachers can partner with families to improve the education and lives of children by doing home visits; holding informal meetings, family–educator meetings, and workshops; volunteering in the classroom; doing special projects; and using electronic communication.

Home Visits

Ideally, an educator's initial contact with families is during a home visit before or at the start of the child's attendance in their program. The policy statement on family engagement (HHS & ED 2016, 15) states that "academic success is associated with trusting relationships between teachers and families that are established at the beginning of the school year through home visits." Home visits are a wonderful way to get to know children and families in their own familiar environment.

For many families, their home turf is their first choice of meeting settings. They don't need to devote time and money to travel to and from the program or find a babysitter. On the other hand, some families are nervous about bringing educators into their home. The chaos in one's life is often reflected in living arrangements, and families may feel they are being judged. In addition, some children may be temporarily living in a foster home, and some children are homeless. Be sensitive to parental concerns and wishes. If you sense reluctance or push-back from families, ask if they would prefer meeting in a neutral place such as a library or community center or even at the program instead of in the family home.

Home visits are encouraged, though, because they offer a unique opportunity to get to know a child where the child can be the host. This gives the child a sense of power, something not often afforded to children, especially if they have a background that includes trauma. It also eases children's anxiety about meeting their teacher for the first time in the school setting or having to compete with other children for introductory time with their educator. In addition, it gives the educator a chance to meet and know children in advance and learn what their favorite toys, foods, and activities are as well as how family members interrelate with one another. This is valuable information for starting the year off on the right foot.

If your program does not support home visits, substitute family–educator meetings. While these meetings provide nearly the same information gleaned from a home visit, home visits are always recommended, primarily because they support bonding both with the child and family members.

Informal Meetings at Arrival and Departure Times

Drop-off and pickup times offer opportunities to have twice-daily conversations with family members who accompany the child to and from the program. More than anything else, these informal meetings can help educators and families forge and strengthen bonds. By seeing each other face to face every day, a relationship is built cumulatively.

When educators greet family members by name and ask about their evening or weekend and how their child is doing, they get to know each other on a personal basis. By listening attentively as family members share or ask questions, they gain each other's trust. These are also good times to share positive anecdotes about children, ask questions, and schedule more formal meetings. At departure, educators can offer family members books and projects they might want to use with their children at home and handouts that will keep families apprised of what children are learning at the program. Some programs have optional take-home kits ready to go, and families can decide if they would like to take one home.

Knowing the benefit in these informal meetings, some programs try to extend the times beyond the 5 or 10 minutes that drop-off and pickup normally take. For example, one child development center holds two-hour coffee hours on Friday mornings, where coffee and donuts are available. Families can use this time to catch up with staff and other enrolled children's family members at a more in-depth, participatory level.

Having built this daily relationship, parents will feel less uptight and threatened when it's time to hold a formal meeting. When families already know their child's educator and trust that they have positive feelings about their child and them, the veneer that trauma builds can be cracked.

Family–Educator Meetings

Regular family–educator meetings (sometimes referred to as parent–teacher conferences) promote in-depth discussions about the children's experiences, progress, and future plans. These meetings are opportunities for educators to share anecdotes and examples of children's learning progress and to raise concerns and seek parental support. They also provide a chance for families to talk about their concerns and support needs with the teacher.

For families of children exposed to trauma, these meetings serve several important purposes that extend beyond the program. Perhaps most importantly, they help educators connect to families and gain the parents' trust that they have their child's—and the family's—best interests at heart. In addition, these meetings let families know how the child is healing and becoming whole.

Here are some tips for conducting effective family–educator conferences:

> Schedule meetings at convenient times for family members. You may need to hold meetings during evenings, before regular work hours, or even on weekends to accommodate attendees' work schedules.

> Before meetings, provide clear communication about timing, attendees, topics, and the family's rights. Give families parking or transportation information, and let them know whether babysitting is available, and whether food will be shared.

> Develop a meeting agenda in advance that is flexible enough to accommodate topics that come up during the meeting. Since children's progress is the focus of meetings, gather all observational information, assessment data, and the child's portfolio to share with families at the meeting. Consider summarizing all the information into a one-page fact sheet that families can take home with them.

> Choose a comfortable, distraction-free area to conduct the conference. Make sure there are adult-sized chairs for all participants so that everyone is comfortable. Avoid sitting behind a desk opposite family members so as not to give the impression that you are in charge and will be doing all the talking.

> Greet family members by name and offer them coffee, tea, or water to set everyone at ease. You want families to feel your warmth and respect and know from the outset that this will be a collaborative session, not one in which they will have to fight for their rights or their child's rights.

> Keep cultural considerations in mind. Maintain an appropriate distance from parents that is typical in their culture. If they do not speak English and you do not speak their home language, arrange for a staff person or interpreter who speaks the language to attend the meeting as well. Let the family know before the meeting that you have made this arrangement.

> Start the conference with a positive anecdote about the child that also compliments the parents. From the start, you want to use the same strengths-based approach with families that you use with children: "First off, I'd like to thank you for making sure Rainbow gets to school on time like we discussed at our last meeting. I don't think she's been late to school a single day this month. Having her be here on time keeps her from being singled out as always late and allows her to be a part of our morning meeting, which is very important educationally and socially. I think being at that meeting has made her days go smoother. So thank you very much for making that happen."

> Focus on jointly promoting the child's healing, resilience, development, and learning. Pause frequently to allow family members to ask questions and make comments. If family members are hesitant to talk, solicit their questions by asking questions such as "What have you noticed at home?" or "Can you tell me what your experiences are?" or "Do you see things differently?"

> Work with the children's families to plan what you should focus on to help the child best develop and succeed. What progress has been made, and where has progress been stalled? What can you do to accelerate progress across all goals? Do other professionals need to be consulted or called in for observation or intervention? Then jointly come up with revised goals that both you and the families feel are most important to concentrate on next. As you set goals, plan with families how they will work with their children at home to complement what is being taught at the program. Perhaps you will need to share classroom materials or reference books with them that will help them work toward the children's goals at home.

Prepare handouts related to the topics you are discussing at the meetings. For example, in Appendix 3, there are several handouts you can reproduce and give to family members to use at home as appropriate.

> End the meeting on a positive note, citing how helpful the parents' cooperation and participation have been. Reiterate that you are all in this together with the common goal of helping their child heal and flourish. They need to know that you see them as assets to their child's progress and that you truly value and are working hard to achieve a strong partnership with them.

Some programs call this approach a compliment sandwich. You begin the meeting with a positive anecdote, discuss the issues, and end with a positive summary. The meeting is thus sandwiched between positives.

As you walk family members out, clarify plans for follow-up from both of you and acknowledge your intent to communicate regularly.

Workshops

Workshops are typically a forum for presenting information of interest to families. Many families view workshops as an opportunity to gain knowledge that will make them more effective parents. For families with children who have experienced trauma, workshops can give them a boost of knowledge, skills, and confidence to help them help their children recover and prosper.

For programs, workshops are a way to embrace families and respond to their needs. Ideally, the topics presented in workshops come by surveying families to learn their preferences for subject matter. Workshops can focus on anything from how trauma affects children's learning to how to handle family stress. You can invite experts to present specialized topics of interest to bring credibility to the presentations and to attract participation.

Planning for these gatherings is similar to preparing for parent–educator conferences. Schedule workshops at times families can easily attend, and find out what supports they might need, like child care or transportation. Arrange to meet these needs, then publicize the workshops well in advance using flyers, emails to families, the program's website, and word of mouth. If needed, a translator should be present.

Volunteering and Participating in Special Projects

Since the first days of Head Start in 1965, family members have been active participants in early childhood program activities. Having parents make presentations and conduct activities is beneficial for the program, the family members who participate, and especially for the children.

Family volunteerism enriches programs by using the talents and skills of family members who bring their cultural and individual practices and ideas to the table. It allows educators to learn more about the children's families and how to embed a family's traditions into programming. It benefits family members by increasing their skill sets as they learn such things as how to best lead a group song with children or accompany the group on a nature walk. It further gives parents confidence in their parenting skills and an opportunity to share their passions and skills with others. However, children benefit the most, as they take pride in having their family members be a part of their education and serve as special members of their class.

Family volunteer participation can take various forms. Most parents enjoy working directly with their child or a small group—reading a book aloud, leading a cooking activity of a favorite family recipe, helping children plant a garden, doing a woodworking project, or helping children put on a puppet show.

To make these activities successful, educators should first let parent volunteers know and understand how these activities work best and provide any helpful training. For example, before coming in to read a group a storybook, most parents appreciate knowing where they should sit in relation to the other children, how they should go through the book, the types of questions to ask, and what to do if children lose interest. To do this, share some of the tips and ideas from Chapter 5 in the section "Choose Books that Will Benefit Children with Trauma Experience." The goal is not just for parents to successfully read a book aloud, but for them to feel good about the experience and to transfer these skills to their home life with their children.

No matter how encouraging or enthusiastic an educator is, some family members may be unable to volunteer in the classroom or family child care program because of work schedules or because insecurities make them hesitant. Parents who have experienced trauma may have their own set of fears about being in the program with children. Educators should meet one on one with these family members to address their concerns and tailor a way for them to participate in the program that will not trigger any of their own fears.

One way to give family members who are reluctant or unable to volunteer a chance to be a part of the program without having to work directly with children is to encourage them to participate in special projects that can be done on their own schedule. This can draw family members in and provide a way for them to contribute to the program. Some ideas for special projects that make use of family members' talents and interests are

> Translating books and song lyrics into the children's home languages

> Recording books and music for children to listen to on headphones

> Making recipe cards of the children's favorite recipes in both English and the children's home languages

> Making prop boxes for dramatic play

> Gathering loose parts for scientific exploration

> Making maracas, tambourines, drums, and other homemade instruments for music and movement

> Making sensory materials for the calming center, such as the glitter jars described in Appendix 3. Directions for making other calming materials can be found on YouTube. Searching for "rainbow sensory bottle" is a good beginning point for finding homemade projects that will help children de-stress. Family members can also make these same materials to use with their children at home.

By working together with families who volunteer in the classroom and on special projects, you can make concrete progress in both forming a working relationship with families and jointly working on mastering the goals you and the children's families have agreed upon for children.

Using Technology to Share Information with Families about Their Children

Technology makes it easy to keep in contact with families. For some parents who find face-to-face contact stressful, staying in touch electronically has many benefits. Among the many ways to communicate electronically with families are the following (Koralek, Nemeth, & Ramsey 2019; Washington 2017):

> **Texts and emails:** Educators can share information easily and instantaneously with families via text and email messages. Depending on each family's preferences, set up a regular schedule and method for connecting. During these electronic check-ins, discuss children's progress, encourage families to raise any concerns, and review plans. This is an opportunity to show parents daily growth and challenges, so there are no surprises when formal meetings occur.

With parental approval, send family members photos and videos of their child engaging in play activities. Nothing makes a parent prouder than seeing their child doing something new or special or even just looking happy. It also will make them appreciate the program staff for being so thoughtful. Be careful, though, not to include any other children in these photos and videos without permission from the parents of those children.

Encourage family members to email or text you if they have concerns or want to discuss something. These written records provide an electronic trail that can be used to track children's progress and ensure you are responding to family members' needs.

If parents have no access to either a smartphone, tablet, or computer, arrange for them to use a public computer or device at the local library near their home or at their work. Sometimes programs will have loaner tablets for families who need one. Phone calls can always be used as a backup method.

> **Photo-based newsletters:** Some educators like to keep families informed with weekly or monthly newsletters. Newsletters can contain such items as a photo-illustrated review of the children's activities (using only photos of children whose families have given permission to publish photos of their children), a portrait of children's social and emotional interactions, snack and mealtime menus, requests for volunteer assistance, and reminders of upcoming field trips or visitors to the program.

Educators might also write short, informative articles about topics such as how the children are learning problem-solving techniques so they can positively resolve conflicts. These feature stories might inspire some reluctant family members to become more involved in the program.

Communication, desktop publishing, and web-based software enables educators to produce professional-looking newsletters with photographs. However, remember the purpose of the newsletter is to share information. It does not need to be elaborate or take up too much of your time to create. Newsletters can be distributed to families in print or via email at the family's preference.

> **Website or Instagram:** Instead of a newsletter, consider creating a class or family child care program website or Instagram account. These platforms can keep families informed through stories, photos, and videos of daily happenings at the program. You may also choose to partner with other online classrooms or family child care programs to become "webpals."

Since photos or videos you use will be posted online, parental approval is mandatory. Carefully review site security settings to prevent posts from being viewed by an unintended audience.

> **Blogs:** Depending on time and interest, educators might also start a blog about life at their program. A blog presents an opportunity to share personal thoughts as an educator with families. For confidentiality reasons, focus the blog on factual information about the program, while still telling stories with humor and personality. Be mindful of posting anything that might upset a parent, colleague, or supervisor, so think about who will be reading these posts before publishing them.

For variety, you might ask the children to dictate stories to you and feature the stories on the blog. Another approach is to have family members author blog posts, featuring perhaps a "Fridays with Families" blog entry.

Sites such as education.weebly.com and blogger.com offer templates for educational blogs and tips for designing your blog. Some of these sites will connect educators to fellow early childhood bloggers around the world.

You may find it advantageous to make use of websites that provide one-stop electronic family engagement, such as ReadyRosie and Kaymbu. They allow you to easily send messages, newsletters, photos, stories, emergency alerts, daily attendance and calendar, children's portfolios of work, and observations and assessments directly to family members through one application. Some sites also provide translation services. Many allow family members to send photos and write-ups back to you, and some, like www. storypark.com, will (with parental permission) allow therapists to join the communication and include their own photos and information about children.

Check with your administrator to see if they use or plan to use one of these all-in-one communication sites specifically designed for educator–family communications. Some of these sites are free. Many offer more robust services for a fee. Most offer free online training.

If your school or program does not use a communication system with built-in design and posting capabilities, help with these functions is available from websites such as education.weebly. com, Shutterfly.com, or educatorpages.com.

With all these technology-based forms of communication, use everyday language that avoids jargon, be respectful, and use gender-neutral language when possible. For families who speak a home language other than English, if you are not fluent in the families' home languages, use a translator or a translator app, or the translation service offered on some of the all-in-one communication systems.

In addition to getting family members' permission to share their child's image and work online, educators must confirm that the program's privacy policies and those of any communication systems being used comply with the Children's Online Privacy Protection Act (COPPA 2020). For further guidance on children's privacy and online safety, consult the policy statements compiled by the Technology in Early Childhood Center at Erikson Institute (Tec Center 2017).

Finally, use school or program accounts for all electronic communication with families. This both protects educators and maintains privacy for families. This caveat applies to all forms of social media. To avoid possible fallout, keep your personal accounts personal. Should your school have a Facebook page or Instagram account, work with your administrator to establish guidelines for contributing to them.

A Path Forward

Connecting with families has been proven to enhance the work educators do with children (Koralek, Nemeth, & Ramsey 2019). For families who have been personally affected by trauma, you will also be helping them heal. The strong relationship you have with parents can help the whole family recover and thrive. This connection may bring rewards that are beyond measure.

In Chapter 9, the healing-centered work you do with children and families will be presented in the context of TIC in schools and communities.

CHAPTER Nine

Trauma-Informed Care in Schools and Communities

Truly effective trauma-informed practice moves beyond what you as an individual can do and encompasses all the other influences in a child's life. It is like a ripple in a pond. The child is at the center, and the rings moving outward are the child's family, you and other staff the child interacts with the most, the rest of your program setting, and the surrounding community.

In other chapters we discussed how to adjust your own practice to create a trauma-informed program that best serves children and how to work with the children's families to support this work. In this chapter we will focus on the school community. The term *school* in this chapter encompasses the community surrounding your learning environment: you, your fellow teachers, your administrator, and all other staff, which may include food service staff, custodians, bus drivers, a school nurse, a librarian, specialists, and guidance counselors. All are members of the school community, and all share responsibility for one another, provide an environment where children can heal and learn, and create a social atmosphere of wellness where all members of the community are supported. In a family child care setting, this community includes other educators you have built relationships with and supervisors or support systems in your area.

Effective TIC relies on cooperation, which is especially essential for applying school- or community-wide TIC policies. This chapter is for both individual educators and the administrators who work with them. TIC policies must be implemented at all levels within the school and guided by school leaders. The intent of this chapter is to offer resources that can be shared with school decision makers.

TIC and the School Community

When a school embraces TIC, it is not simply individual educators who are putting TIC into practice. Rather, the entire system reorganizes to better support children with a history of trauma. This kind of school

> Provides an environment where healing can occur

> Has staff trained to show care and respect to children while seeking solutions and being supportive

> Is welcoming, affirmative, and safe, not only within individual classrooms but also in the organizational structure of the school, community, district, and region

> Extends the same kind of support to both children and the children's families (Wolpow et al. 2016)

No single educator or staff member can create a true TIC learning environment; it takes a team effort. However, because you are a vital player in this effort, you need to look at the big picture to understand where and how you and your efforts fit in to the overall TIC plan. In addition, you will be able to recognize good practice and support the school as its TIC efforts evolve and expand.

The Four Rs Framework and Six Principles of TIC

To build a program-wide TIC program, a common foundation of information and ability to apply TIC must exist. SAMHSA (2014a) has created a framework for a trauma-informed approach that rests on four key assumptions (the Four Rs) and six key principles. The idea is that if people at every level of the organization understand these concepts, they have a solid foundation for a TIC school. The Four Rs of TIC (SAMHSA 2014a) are

1. **R**ealize the widespread impact of trauma.

2. **R**ecognize the signs of trauma and traumatic response.

3. **R**espond by using the knowledge and resources available to provide TIC.

4. **R**esist re-traumatization of children and staff by consistently evaluating policies and practices to make sure they promote healing and do not inadvertently create more stress. (9)

In addition to having a framework, a trauma-informed approach follows six primary agreed-upon principles of TIC developed by a team of national experts, including trauma survivors (SAMHSA 2014a):

1. Safety

2. Trustworthiness and transparency

3. Peer support

4. Collaboration and mutuality

5. Empowerment, voice, and choice

6. Cultural, historical, and gender issues (10)

School administrators must recognize that staff members at all levels play a role in TIC and that they must emphasize partnering and shared decision making. In "Roles and Responsibilities for Implementing Trauma-Informed Care," on pages 87–88, you can see your role in implementing these principles of TIC along with your school community's responsibility for ensuring that trauma-informed practices are a universal part of your school's practice and culture.

What TIC Looks Like in Action

Following the principles outlined above, schools need to ensure that all staff feel empowered to support children's needs and that everyone actively participates in helping children heal and succeed. If a custodian, for example, notices a child wearing clothes that are inappropriate for the weather, or a teaching assistant notices changes in a child's behavior, they should know that as part of a TIC team, it is their job to discuss these observations with a supervisor. In addition, administrators need to recognize that adding expectations of TIC for educators without providing assistance with other duties is unsustainable. As a school's TIC program is developed, administrators must ensure that opportunities for building and maintaining a TIC practice are ingrained in the school culture.

It is essential for everyone in the school community to focus on strengths-based initiatives that enhance children's abilities. This happens when everyone is aware of the language they use when discussing children in the program, making sure that conversations focus on identifying and affirming strengths rather than dwelling on problems (Wolpow et al. 2016). Consider this example: A lead teacher and teaching assistant are discussing an interaction in a block area where a child is working. When the child's work is disturbed, she lashes out verbally at other children. Rather than saying "Kara is such a problem! She doesn't want anyone else to play in that area. She needs to learn to use her words and be nicer!," they might instead say "Kara was really focused on her block building this morning. It was difficult for her when her concentration was broken by the other children. What can we do to let Kara keep working while also letting other children use the blocks? What are some ways we can help her express what she needs calmly?"

Roles and Responsibilities for Implementing Trauma-Informed Care

TIC Principle	The Educator's Role	The School Community's Policy (SAMHSA 2014a)
Safety	■ Make sure the indoor and outdoor environments are physically safe and hazard-free. ■ Ensure adequate space and adult supervision for play. ■ Create welcoming spaces for families to drop off and pick up children and meet with you. ■ Make sure that only authorized individuals can visit the program and pick up children. ■ Interact with children and families in ways that make them feel safe and valued. ■ Create a predictable daily schedule and let children know if there will be changes. ■ Practice fire, evacuation, and sheltering in place procedures.	Staff, children, and families feel physically and psychologically safe. The physical environment and interpersonal interactions offer safety.
Trustworthiness and transparency	■ Make a conscious effort to form a relationship with each child as a precursor to teaching and learning. ■ Make an intentional effort to form a reciprocal relationship with each family. ■ Regard children's challenging behaviors as trauma related and not attempts to misbehave. ■ Commit to ending punitive actions such as suspension and expulsion. ■ Be clear in tasks, directions, and goals. ■ Respect children's boundaries and sensitivities. ■ Ensure children's and families' confidentiality and privacy practices. ■ Refrain from making promises you can't keep to either children or families.	The goal of school operations and decisions is to gain the trust of children, families, and staff.
Peer support	■ Bring together families to help each other and offer support. ■ To help children identify and resolve their own problems, use anonymous stories you've been given permission to share or anonymous stories of other people who have experienced trauma. ■ Use bibliotherapy to help children process their feelings.	*Peers* refers to children and family members who have experienced trauma. Peers are integral to the school's delivery of services to build trust and establish safety and empowerment. Families and children learn from others who have experienced similar situations.

(continues)

TIC Principle	The Educator's Role	The School Community's Policy (SAMHSA 2014a)
Collaboration and mutuality	■ Strong relationships are key to working with colleagues as well as children and families. ■ Meet with colleagues regularly to brainstorm strategies and approaches. ■ Look to supervisors for guidance and leadership. Invite them and specialists into the class to observe and advise. ■ Work with a specialist, such as the school librarian, if there is one, to select books on trauma and emotions to read with children. ■ Include support staff in programming. ■ Encourage a collaborative environment so that educators who spend more time in one-on-one relationships have support in accomplishing other tasks.	The school recognizes that everyone plays a role in TIC and that healing can happen only through relationships. This helps level power differences and encourage joint decision making.
Empowerment, voice, and choice	■ Use strengths-based teaching that does not focus on perceived deficits. ■ Individualize all programming, valuing the uniqueness of each child and family. ■ Build choice into programming, recognizing that all choices are acceptable. ■ Use a philosophy of "doing with" rather than "doing for" with children and families. ■ Stress realistic optimism with children and families. ■ Offer appropriate praise regularly.	Recognize, build on, and validate children's, families', and staff members' strengths. Maintain an underlying belief in resilience and in the ability to heal from trauma.
Cultural, historical, and gender issues	■ Seek to understand and apply knowledge of cultural, historical, and gender issues in interactions with children and families. ■ Be culturally responsive in policies and classroom choices. ■ Provide responsive services that children and families can access easily.	The school actively moves past cultural stereotypes and biases based on race, ethnicity, sexual orientation, age, religion, gender identity, geography, and so on. The entire school community is aware of historical trauma and the role it plays.

In addition, staff need access to regular training to help them put TIC into practice and to know which resources are available to them. Having a coordinated approach allows you to learn from each other and to be more effective in your teaching and relationship building. These resources will vary from program to program but could include reviewing your daily interactions with children and finding ways to seamlessly integrate positive interactions and shift your approach from reactive to proactive. It could also include meeting with supervisors regularly to discuss children you are concerned about or problems you are having with your teaching and asking them to observe and give you feedback.

Smaller programs may look outside their school for support from others who are in a similar situation. Outside support might include local support groups for faith-based schools, schools with a specialty curriculum, or family child care programs. Organizations like NAEYC or the National Association for Family Child Care (NAFCC) can help you locate a group in your area.

Fall-Hamilton Elementary School in Nashville, Tennessee, uses a tap in/tap out program that allows a teacher to request coverage for their class so they can step out for a short break and regain their composure when needed (Berger 2018). While this may not be practical in all situations, it does illustrate that there are small ways that entire school communities can work together to create a TIC school.

Studies show that for children to thrive, they need a strong, caring relationship with two to three trusted adults in their school or program (Williams with Scherrer 2017). Focusing on growing these relationships is the first step to supporting and strengthening children and allowing them to learn. One suggestion from *Trauma Toolkit* (Williams with Scherrer 2017) is to pass around a list of students' names at a staff meeting or during professional development and ask each staff person to put their initials next to the names of children they feel they have a strong, positive relationship with. To ensure that no child slips through the cracks, staff can put extra effort into connecting with children who have fewer than two or three sets of initials next to their names.

Treat relationships with families with the same care, and reinforce that they are welcomed in small and large ways. Offer information in the languages used by families in your school so they have multiple ways to communicate with staff and be involved in the classroom. Along with other staff, make a deliberate effort to get to know the families.

Strengths and experiences should be recognized and built on, both among staff and with the children and families. Families need to know that their voices matter and their valuable input will be used to create a better environment for their child. Rather than assume they know what is best for a child or the family, everyone in the school must listen and collaborate openly. Actively working to move past stereotypes and biases should be an ongoing process in TIC. This includes respecting cultural connections and historical trauma and ensuring all policies are responsive to the needs of each person.

Trauma-informed educators should not be discouraged when they propose changes they know will benefit students but are met with resistance. In these instances, remember that resistance is often rooted in fear of the unknown. Other educators and staff who are hesitant need to be heard and to have their concerns addressed so they can adjust to the changes.

Circle Preschool Program

The Circle Preschool program in Richmond, Virginia, was launched by Greater Richmond Stop Child Abuse Now (SCAN) in 2015 to offer family-focused, therapeutic early childhood education in Richmond (Price 2018). It provides trauma-informed services to preschoolers who have experienced severe trauma, many of whom have either never been to preschool or were expelled from other programs. It is an example of what the best practices of TIC can look like, and its model can be adapted to other programs.

The program focuses on three Rs: regulate, relate, and reason. Dr. Kathy Ryan explains that the intention is to "help these little ones learn there are safe people in the world," learn how to process and express their intense feelings, and allow them to successfully build and maintain relationships.

Administrators have ensured that Circle Preschool is effective by guaranteeing

- High ratios of trained staff to children

- Classrooms designed to meet children's needs

- Child-informed curricula that incorporate children's interests, developing critical thinking skills, and collaboration and relationship building

- Additional therapeutic aides, an occupational therapist, and other specialists who work with the school

- Close relationships with families, including regular meetings with parents or guardians

Working with Your Administrator

Creating this school-wide focus on TIC means collaborating with others in your school to make necessary changes. Sporleder and Forbes (2016) assert that at least 75 to 80 percent support from the staff and 100 percent support from administration are needed to make lasting, widespread changes and create a TIC school. Administrative support is necessary so that you can make necessary changes to your schedule, learning environment, teaching practice, and so on. Staff support will ensure that there is continuity for children throughout their day.

The administrative support also sets the tone and philosophy for the school so that everyone, including families, knows what the school stands for. In practice, this means making sure that your administration supports staff and students' strengths, identifies and implements professional development opportunities, and provides both in-school and outside resources like mental health professionals and social workers for you and other staff.

In addition, administrators can re-evaluate guidance policies to make them more trauma informed. Leadership can also identify the many services available through local, state, and federal government or community-based social organizations that benefit children, including nutrition programs, support for families experiencing homelessness, and sliding-scale mental health resources. The school can be a valuable hub to coordinate these many resources and help families access them.

As you work with your school leadership to modify your program to become a more trauma-informed school, use the following ideas, based on the Flexible Framework developed by the Massachusetts Advocates for Children (Cole et al. 2005):

> Train staff to recognize trauma and to provide strategies to help children cope, learn, and thrive.

> Review program-wide infrastructure and culture and identify ways to integrate trauma-informed practices into what you are already doing.

An Administrator's Viewpoint on Creating a TIC Program

For Lauren Dotson (2017), an administrator in a pre-K to 8 school, creating a TIC program involved the following:

■ Understanding the "frequent flyers," as Dotson refers to students who were often sent to her for behavior problems, and what was happening in their lives—including traumas—that influenced their behavior.

■ Looking beyond board guidance policies for how to support students. This included collaborating with community agencies to provide services, working across departments to make individual student care plans, and creating a committee of teacher mentors who could help those still learning TIC practices.

■ Encouraging teachers to ask administrators for support rather than just to control behavior. Allowing students to come to them to have a break, helping teachers better distinguish behaviors that needed to be referred for class disruption from those that could be resolved in class.

■ Getting to know children individually and creating a safe haven for them.

> Use relationships your school has developed with local mental health providers, homeless and women's shelters, the department of youth and family services, and other organizations that can support children and families.

> Review your teaching methods for helping children who have experienced trauma.

> Identify other nonacademic ways for supporting children.

> Ensure children have a strong relationship with two or three adults in the program.

> Review school policies (especially guidance) from a trauma-informed lens and adjust them as needed.

> Develop a plan to engage parents, foster parents, resource parents, and guardians as outlined in Chapter 8 and build strong relationships with families.

To ensure that your program is implementing TIC in its intended form and spirit, you may wish to make use of or adapt a checklist such as the "Trauma-Sensitive School Checklist" created by Lesley University and Massachusetts Advocates for Children (see www.tolerance.org).

Ideally, the entire school staff will use the same checklist to ensure high quality across the board. Your administrator and TIC peer groups can brainstorm how best to rectify gaps in the TIC framework. You may find that some items are not relevant to your program.

Advocacy

As an early childhood educator, you are uniquely positioned to not only help individual children and families as they experience and recover from traumatic events but also to advocate for better resources and interventions for the wider community. Help others see that you are advocating for *children,* not victims, and focus on building strengths and achieving successes.

To significantly effect change, communities need resources to eradicate causes of trauma and provide wide-ranging interventions when needed. This won't happen without awareness, changes in legislation and community culture, and resources like parenting education, mental health services, reliable access to medical care, job opportunities, and continuing education and training available to all.

These big challenges can make advocacy seem overwhelming, especially if you think about large movements (federal legislative change, large-scale marches). However, many types of advocacy and awareness can effectively make an impact. You can take the following steps now:

> **Educate yourself:** Become more aware of trauma and TIC. Take steps to ensure you have a trauma-sensitive program and use techniques that support children and families. Continue to read books and magazine articles, attend workshops, and join discussions online or participate in organizations in your area.

> **Educate others:** Share what you learn with co-workers and families. Provide information, resources they can use, and actions they can take. Lead a professional development workshop or parent meeting and contribute to newsletters or communications from your program. If you enjoy writing or participate in social media, share information through newsletters, emails, your program or school website, Facebook, Twitter, or Instagram. The most powerful way to educate others is by sharing your personal story. Talking about how you've seen children and families thrive through resilience and TIC or about your own life experience is incredibly effective for helping people understand the information and, more important, how it applies to real life.

Pair that with information from local, state, and federal organizations that give people the supporting facts. Groups like Voices for Virginia's Children have created short fact sheets that help make the information easier to understand, as shown in Figure 7 on pages 93–94. In this instance, voters can use the fact sheet to determine which potential candidates running for local and state office support TIC. This fact sheet explores issues such as historical trauma and equity. Your state may have similar materials targeted at voters. If it doesn't, consider volunteering to develop one.

> **Support others:** Many child advocacy groups work to support children and families on local, regional, and national levels. Look for a group in your area that is doing work that inspires you and see how you can help. One place to start is with your local or state NAEYC affiliate advocacy branch. Find the branch closest to you at www.naeyc.org /get-involved/membership/affiliates/network.

> **Get engaged:** To make legislative changes, look for training in public policy, such as that offered by the NAEYC Public Policy Forum. Volunteer on boards or committees for child advocacy. An important way to get engaged is to call your state and national members of Congress to ask them to focus on issues related to childhood trauma. Find your elected officials at www.usa.gov/elected-officials or through local advocacy groups. Support election campaigns for candidates who share your ideals, and consider running for an elected position yourself!

A Path Forward

Steps you take to increase awareness of trauma's effects on children and to help more children get the support they need will help to ensure that all children with a trauma history heal and succeed in both school and life.

TRAUMA-INFORMED VIRGINIA

A trauma-informed approach to working with children and families asks "what happened to you?" not "what's wrong with you?" Our policymakers must prioritize preventing trauma, intervening early to address traumatic experiences, and dismantling systems that perpetuate trauma.

— ADVERSE CHILDHOOD EXPERIENCES (ACEs) —

Many children experience trauma, which impacts their brain development and their long-term health and well-being.

 Separation from a parent including death or incarceration

 Living with or experiencing **domestic violence, parental substance abuse** or **mental illness,** or **community violence**

 Physical or **emotional abuse** or **neglect**

 Economic hardship

20% of children in Virginia have experienced two or more ACEs

The best way to buffer the impacts of trauma is to educate and encourage parents to provide safe and nurturing homes.

Early childhood home visiting programs provide support to pregnant women and families with children ages 0 to 5

but only reach 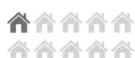 **<10%** of families in need

Too often the professionals who work with children and families experience burnout related to job stressors.

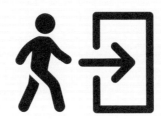 **50%** of child welfare workers **thought about leaving their positions if offered a less stressful job**

Trauma experienced by some children and families is layered on top of racial or historical trauma.

RACIAL TRAUMA & HISTORICAL TRAUMA

RACIAL TRAUMA
The stressful impact or emotional pain of one's experience with racism and discrimination

HISTORICAL TRAUMA
Cumulative emotional and psychological harm, as a result of group traumatic experiences, transmitted across generations within communities and families

Figure 7. Fact sheet on trauma for Virginia voters. Reprinted, by permission, from Voices for Virginia's Children, "2019 Election Guide," 9–10. https://vakids.org/wp-content/uploads/2019/08/2019-VVC-Election_Toolkits_ALL_WEB.pdf.

(continues)

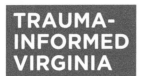

Questions for Candidates

#VAVotes4Kids

1 **TRAUMA-INFORMED SCHOOLS:** The Virginia School Safety Audit Report noted that half of the threat assessments made in schools were for self-harm. Teachers are reporting an increase of children with challenging behaviors, most often linked to trauma experienced at home or in the community. **What would you do to ensure that teachers and school divisions have the resources to meet their children's socio-emotional and mental health needs?**

2 **CROSS-SYSTEM COLLABORATION:** Children can interact with many systems (schools, health and mental health, courts) as they grow up. At times these systems do not work together and can create additional challenges for families. **What would you do to ensure better outcomes for children and families involved in multiple systems?**

3 **MENTAL HEALTH IN SCHOOLS:** To begin to address students' mental health needs, the General Assembly added more school counselor positions. These positions are considered "support staff along with nurses, social workers, and school psychologists. **Do you believe that schools have adequate support staff? Why or why not?**

4 **ACCESS TO CARE:** Virginia policymakers are presented with two opportunities to implement more trauma-informed and evidence-based initiatives for children and their families; the implementation of the Family First Prevention Services Act in foster care and the redesign of Medicaid-funded behavioral health initiatives. This process will require scaling-up services, training staff, and data collection and evaluation. **What do you hope will be better for vulnerable children and their families after the roll-out of these initiatives?**

5 **COMMUNITY-LEVEL PREVENTION:** Over 20 communities across Virginia are forming regional trauma-informed networks to foster trauma prevention and facilitate trauma-informed practices in health, courts, schools, and other systems. **What role, if any, should the state play in advancing these efforts?**

6 **WORKFORCE:** Child-serving professionals including teachers, mental health professionals, and social workers are reporting high job stress and vicarious or secondary trauma from working with children who have experienced trauma. **What efforts would you champion to support these professionals?**

7 **EQUITY + TRAUMA:** Historical policy decisions, such as school segregation, have led to decades of negative consequences for generations of families and neighborhoods. For some children their ACEs are layered on top of these historical traumas. **Are there policy solutions that can address both the historical and current effects of trauma? If so, what are they?**

CHAPTER Ten   Caring for Yourself

This book is about healing and hope. For children. For the children's families. And for you, the early childhood educator. Trauma touches everyone. If left unchecked, it is likely to leave harm in its wake. That is why you must be vigilant and proactive, both with those you work with and yourself. In this chapter, we focus on how to prevent the ill effects of trauma from creeping into your own life. The self-care strategies highlighted here will help you remain strong and healthy enough to be the champion for children and families with a history of trauma that you want and need to be.

Self-care may not be the first thing that comes to mind when most people think of dealing with trauma. As an educator, your focus is first and foremost on the children you teach. You also work with family members to support children's learning goals and consult with specialists, team with colleagues, meet with supervisors, and interact with members of the community. You devote a lot of time, energy, and professional responsibilities to many other people, but you may not devote enough time to yourself.

Being an early childhood educator can be both physically and mentally exhausting. Preschoolers and kindergartners are whirlwinds of energy, exploring, experimenting, and making discoveries. They depend on you to put them first, meeting their needs, and helping them attain their aspirations. At the same time, they bring joy as you see them mastering tasks, learning new concepts, and appreciating you for being such an important part of their lives. But there is no denying they can drain you of energy and leave you feeling spent.

When you add trauma to the equation, the chances that you will sometimes feel overwhelmed and find it difficult to go on increase dramatically. Children who have experienced trauma, as you have been reading and perhaps experiencing in your own program, often respond to it in ways that test your patience and push you to the limit. Children who are in survival mode can be aggressive, rude, uncooperative, and inattentive. And until you help children feel calm and safe and learn to self-regulate, you cannot focus on other kinds of learning.

Your Own Compounding Stress

If you have endured the same traumatic experiences as the children—a natural disaster, school violence, or national crises such as the COVID-19 pandemic—you may share similar fight-flight-freeze responses in your own life. You may be dealing with issues like the loss of personal property or even grieving over the injury or death of a loved one. Like a number of early childhood educators, you may also be a survivor of your own childhood traumas, which may or may not have been resolved. Hearing of the children's experiences and fears can bring back unhappy memories that temporarily paralyze or haunt you.

Moreover, if your program or home is in a neighborhood characterized by violence or poverty, you are likely to experience the same ongoing traumas as the children you care for and teach. For you and them, traumas are an ongoing concern.

The early childhood profession can itself be a source of financial stress. Despite the recognized importance of early education to children's lives, it is among the lowest-paying fields (Nicholson et al. 2020). Many early childhood teachers work supplemental jobs to earn a living wage. And even with frequent moonlighting, early childhood educators use government subsidies at more than double the rate of workers across all occupations (Austin et al. 2019).

The economic stresses of being an early childhood professional are felt hardest by women of color. Early childhood teachers are almost exclusively women, and unlike the K–12 and postsecondary educational sectors, where 75 percent of teachers are White, the early care and education sector comprises 40 percent people of color (Austin et al. 2019). In addition, Black and Latino early childhood educators are more likely to have the lower-paying assistant teacher jobs than are White educators. These circumstances have led the Center for the Study of Child Care Employment to proclaim, "The current early education system is built on racial inequities" (Austin et al. 2019).

All of these pressures can put chronic stress on you. Before you even begin your day with young children, you may already be feeling the economic squeeze of low wages and perhaps prejudice and racism as well. The selflessness it takes to work with, nurture, and teach young children is testament to the commitment those who have chosen this profession have.

The good news is that you can take action to counteract your own stress. This chapter explores the range of stress-related conditions early childhood educators may experience and offers practical ideas you can implement right away to ease the stress of your job. Stress does not have to take a toll when self-care is a priority. As the saying goes, you need to be well to do well. And by doing so, you can position yourself to enjoy teaching's many rewards.

Defining Teaching-Related Stress

As society has learned more about trauma and its effects, researchers have begun to look at how educators who work with young children with trauma are affected by the experience. In doing so, they have defined and delineated how stress-related manifestations are triggered, what the symptoms are, and how they can be treated.

Burnout

Burnout is probably the best known of these phenomena. Burnout is "a reaction to prolonged or chronic job stress [that] is characterized by three main dimensions: exhaustion, cynicism (less identification with the job), and feelings of reduced professional ability" (Freudenberger & Richelson 1980). Burnout can bring about physical, psychological, cognitive, and relational disturbances (Nicholson et al. 2020; Transitional Support, n.d.).

While you may experience work-related burnout, it is not directly tied to working with children with trauma. Rather, it is the cumulative effect of general occupational stress and is not related to the emotional toll of hearing about and helping children overcome trauma. However, burnout can sometimes occur in combination with secondary trauma conditions.

Secondary trauma conditions that stem from absorbing the impacts of others' trauma go by several names: *secondary traumatic stress*, *compassion fatigue*, and *vicarious traumatization* (Bride, Radey, & Figley 2007). *Empathy fatigue*, *empathic distress*, and *empathy distress fatigue* are newer terms for health problems brought on by stress (Alber 2018). Although these conditions are all related, and many are alternate names for the same conditions, some nuances should be distinguished.

Secondary Traumatic Stress/Compassion Fatigue

Secondary traumatic stress (STS) is the term most commonly found in the literature to describe the phenomenon brought on by helping someone exposed to trauma. Anyone involved in empathically listening to the trauma stories of children and their families is vulnerable to developing this condition. It takes only one indirect exposure to traumatic material to be affected. Hearing about the traumatic event—not experiencing it—causes the reaction.

The National Child Traumatic Stress Network describes the condition this way (NCTSN 2011):

> Secondary traumatic stress is the emotional duress that results when an individual hears about the firsthand trauma experiences of another. Its symptoms mimic those of PTSD. . . . Individuals affected by secondary stress may find themselves re-experiencing personal trauma or notice an increase in arousal and avoidance reactions related to the indirect trauma exposure. They may also experience changes in memory and perception; alterations in their sense of self-efficacy; a depletion of personal resources; and disruption in their perceptions of safety, trust, and independence. (2)

A more recent and popular term is *compassion fatigue,* often perceived as a kinder, less stigmatizing way to describe this phenomenon. According to the NCTSN (2011) and the ACF (n.d.), the terms *STS* and *compassion fatigue* are interchangeable and refer to the same condition. In this book, we will refer to all secondary stress as compassion fatigue.

While the symptoms of compassion fatigue vary from individual to individual, they most typically involve empathic drain and chronic exhaustion. Other PTSD-like symptoms might include fear, guilt, anxiety, apathy, sense of hopelessness, sleep disturbances, nightmares and intrusive thoughts, hypervigilance, short temperedness, and a denial of problems. These symptoms can further express themselves in compulsive behaviors (overspending, overeating, gambling) and drug use to mask feelings (ACF, n.d. a; Compassion Fatigue Awareness Project, n.d.; Gunn, n.d.; NCTSN 2011; Nicholson et al. 2020).

Everyone who teaches children with a trauma background is susceptible to developing compassion fatigue. Many believe it is an inevitable consequence of being a caring individual. Some early childhood educators, however, are more likely to develop compassion fatigue than others: women, new teachers, those who are most empathic by nature, and those who have their own unresolved personal trauma (NCTSN 2011; Ollison 2019).

Empathy Fatigue/Empathic Distress/Empathy Distress Fatigue

Other terms for the condition of compassion fatigue use the word *empathy.* Halifax, who first adopted the term *empathic distress,* uses these terms "to describe what happens when someone is exposed repeatedly to the trauma of others. . . . For teachers, that feeling of deep empathy for a student, coupled with knowing that you've done all you can do—and the child is still perhaps still suffering—can cause considerable distress" (Alber 2018, 2).

All empathy-related terms can be used interchangeably and as substitutes for the terms *secondary traumatic stress* and *compassion fatigue.* Proponents of these empathy-related terms argue that since empathy is at the root of this stress-related condition, it is more accurate to use an empathy-related term to describe that connection. For now, though, compassion fatigue remains the more popular and accepted term.

Vicarious Trauma

Vicarious trauma also results from empathic engagement with children who have experienced trauma. This type of trauma can be described as "the emotional residue of exposure that [educators] have from working with people as they are hearing their trauma stories and become witnesses to the pain, fear, and terror that trauma survivors have endured" (American Counseling Association 2011).

What distinguishes vicarious trauma from compassion fatigue is that vicarious trauma leads to cognitive disruptions that have a long-lasting impact on one's personal beliefs and world view (Quitangon 2019). This type of trauma response hits at the heart of your essence. It typically disrupts what makes you you—eating away at your sense of hope, spirituality, and meaning of life (Office of Justice Programs, n.d.).

Those who develop vicarious trauma typically overreact to events and project cynicism and pessimism. The condition not only influences what happens in the workplace but also has serious repercussions on an educator's personal life and relationships. Those with vicarious trauma tend to experience a loss of purpose and joy (American Counseling Association 2011; Transitional Support, n.d.).

However, just as it is possible to overturn the signs of compassion fatigue, it is possible through self-care to develop resilience from vicarious trauma. You can even achieve what is known as *vicarious transformation*—an ability to find compassion satisfaction in work and restored meaning in life (Office of Justice Programs, n.d.).

Using Self-Care to Overcome Secondary Trauma

If you experience secondary trauma, you are not alone. Even if you have no signs of compassion fatigue or vicarious trauma now, that doesn't mean you are immune to developing one of these conditions. Stress can be cumulative. In addition, as situations change, stress levels fluctuate. The more you can attend to your own well-being now, the better you will weather whatever stressors arise later.

None of this reflects poorly on you or is something to be ashamed of. And it certainly doesn't mean that you're not a good teacher. To the contrary, those who experience compassion fatigue and vicarious trauma do so because they are deeply empathic and take children's traumas to heart. All early childhood educators need to know this because it can happen to anyone and, most important, it can be effectively addressed.

Successfully treating and overcoming the symptoms of compassion fatigue and vicarious trauma is a two-step process: 1) make yourself aware that you have the condition and acknowledge it, and 2) make self-care an integral part of your routine. Though seemingly easy to do, these can be difficult tasks for many educators who feel they do not have the time or resources to care for themselves.

Awareness

Once you understand the signs and symptoms of secondary trauma presented in this chapter, take them seriously. You might ask a colleague to help you assess your stress levels and share your thoughts with each other so that you each have an outside opinion. If you or a colleague suspects that being surrounded by trauma is affecting you, that should be your call to action.

To out find out how your work is affecting you both positively and negatively, consider searching online for the Professional Quality of Life Measure (ProQOL). This free 30-item questionnaire measures not only compassion fatigue, vicarious trauma, and burnout but also *compassion satisfaction*. This term can be defined as "the pleasure you derive from being able to do your work well" (Hudnall Stamm 2009). It refers to the positive feelings that characterize the work you do with children and the sense of fulfillment you experience in seeing children heal and thrive. Compassion satisfaction is most likely why you became a teacher in the first place. It's what you want to achieve so that you are not only successful in the work you do but also proud of your success.

Remember, though, that results from an online quiz are not a substitute for a clinical diagnosis. This quiz will give you insight and help guide you as you decide which self-care options you should take. If you have concerns, though, talk with a qualified mental health professional.

Awareness will lead you to step two—taking action. Even if you feel that your risk of secondary trauma is currently low, it is still highly recommended that you use self-care as a preventive health measure.

Self-Care Strategies

Self-care is often categorized as self-indulgence. Many people regard it as pampering used by those without the self-discipline to "get on with things." Even those who don't think of self-care as selfish or wasteful frequently regard it as a low-priority or luxury activity.

Yet, self-care is basic to our everyday existence. "Self-care is the 'oxygen' that keeps us alive, healthy, and functioning at our best capacity. Self-care is BREATH!" (Grise-Owens 2019). Rather than view self-care as self-indulgence, try reframing it as self-respect.

Self-care involves incorporating activities aimed at restoring and improving your physical and emotional well-being into your everyday life. The NCTSN (2011) recommends focusing on cognitive-behavioral and mindfulness-based strategies for best results.

Listed below are 15 strategies targeted to help you heal from secondary stress and to fortify you for the future. Strategies 1, 5, 11, and 15 are considered integral to recovery and are starred. They have been recognized in the research literature as contributing to wellness, particularly in combatting compassion fatigue. When setting goals for yourself, we therefore suggest that you begin with these items. From the remaining 11 strategies, choose those that most appeal to you and that you are most likely to use habitually.

Make the strategies you select a part of your daily life. Most people find it helpful to start slowly. Begin with two or three strategies. Once they become routine, start adding others.

Strategy 15 helps you turn your personal self-care goals into an action plan. Charting your goals and monitoring your progress will help ensure that you are on a steady course toward compassion satisfaction.

*1. Be kind to yourself.

This strategy could be called *respect yourself* because tending to your basic wellness needs should not be a favor or privilege you extend yourself but something you do every day to be your healthiest and best-functioning self. As a kindness to yourself and those you work with, attend to your physical, social, mental, emotional, and spiritual needs as best you can (Scott 2019). Here are some suggestions:

> **Physical needs:** Regularly eat nutritiously balanced meals; sleep adequately; exercise regularly; monitor and attend to your health needs, making and keeping needed doctor and dental appointments and taking any medications as prescribed.

> **Social needs:** Cultivate and maintain close friendships. Everyone has different social needs, but we all need to share others' company in some capacity. Determine what your needs are and build time into your schedule to have face-to-face time with your friends that feels right for you.

> **Mental health needs:** Do activities to keep your mind sharp, such as work crosswords and other puzzles, read books, or research something you are interested in and passionate about. To be mentally healthy, you also need to be proactive. If you feel depressed, anxious, or otherwise troubled, talk about it with a doctor or therapist. (See Strategy 14 for more on this topic.) Treatment can make a world of difference.

> **Emotional needs:** Establish appropriate ways to process your emotions. Talk to someone close to you—a spouse, partner, relative, or friend—to air your feelings and talk problems through. Journal your feelings; seeing things written out sometimes gives a different slant to events. (See Strategy 9 for more on journaling.) Exercise, take baths, or spend time doing hobbies (see Strategy 10) that allow you to relax and refocus, such as painting. Remember that alcohol and other drugs can suppress your feelings rather than help you manage and lessen your distress. They may even intensify your emotional or physical pain.

> **Spiritual needs:** Nurturing your spirit involves doing things that bring meaning to your life and a connection with the world. It doesn't have to involve religion, although it certainly can. Build in time for praying, meditating (see Strategy 5), or volunteering for a cause that enriches your soul (see Strategy 8).

2. Get good at the balancing game.

It's not always easy to turn off your thoughts about the important work you do once you leave for the day. To make your life less stressful, boundaries are needed. Challenge yourself to do the following:

> Leave your program on time one or two days a week.

> Leave your teacher bag at the program one or two days a week.

> Exercise directly after leaving the program.

> Treat yourself to something special once a month—a manicure, a special coffee, or a movie, for instance.

Once you make these actions a habit, try increasing the number of days a week you leave work on time without your teaching materials. Eventually this will become a habit. Try to use your time away from the program to focus on family, friends, and yourself. Being able to spend more energy on your family is bound to help repair the problems characteristic of compassion fatigue and vicarious trauma. And feeling better at home will energize you to be a better educator when you are at work.

3. Practice time management.

Time management is related to adding balance to your life. Allot specific times in your daily calendar for work, family, social life, personal needs, chores, and pleasure, including alone time. Blocking time allows you to know in advance when you should gear things down and prepare to refocus on another activity. To see if you are comfortable with the way your day flows, take an online time management quiz.

4. Assert yourself appropriately.

It may sound like an odd self-care technique to stand up for your rights, needs, and wishes in ways that are respectful of both yourself and others. However, assertiveness, when appropriate, can increase your confidence, self-efficacy, and personal agency—all of which will help you feel less stressed and better about yourself and your work. Asserting yourself reduces stress and anger, promotes competence and the respect of others, and improves decision-making and coping skills (Mayo Clinic 2017).

Learn to say no. Because you work in a helping profession, you may feel obligated to be there when someone wants something from you—even when doing so is not in your best interests. Carol Rickard (2018), a "stressologist," suggests that you regard your "no muscle" as you would a real muscle and realize that the more you exercise it, the stronger it will become. She suggests acknowledging both your desire and regret: "I would love to help; I am just not able to." Or, "I wish I could, however, I can't change my appointment."

Many methods of addressing aggressiveness involve both spoken and body language. Remember that appropriate assertiveness is based on balance; aggressiveness is based on winning. Keep these pointers in mind (Mayo Clinic 2017; Taylor 2013):

> Value yourself, your rights, and your needs. Show self-confidence, but not self-importance.

> Make eye contact when you talk with others. This shows your interest in them and your desire to have two-way communication.

> Use posture to convey body language that carries the messages you want to send. Experts suggest adopting an upright and relaxed posture and leaning forward slightly toward the other person without infringing on their personal space. Try to maintain a neutral or positive facial expression. Practice how you want to convey your body language in front of a mirror or ask a friend or colleague to critique how you present yourself.

> Avoid being accusatory by using "I" statements. Rather than saying to someone, "You're wrong," try saying, "I disagree." Instead of telling someone, "You make me angry," try saying, "I feel frustrated."

> Wait a bit before talking if you feel overly emotional. Give yourself time to calm down, so you don't become angry or frustrated.

> Start where it's safe. Practice being more appropriately assertive in low-risk situations such as with a spouse or close friend. Once you feel more comfortable, branch out to others. Eventually try your new communication skills at work, where more is on the line, including potential rewards.

*5. Cultivate mindfulness.

Just as mindfulness can help children recover from trauma and better connect to their educators, it can also help adults overcome the impacts of compassion fatigue and vicarious trauma. In fact, mindfulness is recognized as one of the most successful strategies for counteracting the effects of compassion fatigue (NCTSN 2011).

Mindfulness modulates the structure of the brain (Manitoba Trauma Information & Education Centre, n.d. a). Over time, mindfulness practices build connections and slow down reactivity. Similar to what happens with children, through these changes in brain architecture, you develop increased emotional regulation and the ability to tolerate emotional challenges. The effects of mindfulness extend your ability to better accept professional and personal frustrations with relationships.

Mindfulness can also improve your work with children because it strengthens the part of your brain associated with interpreting emotions and allows you to compassionately experience others' feelings, which enhances empathy. Educators who practice mindfulness have more positive teaching experiences than educators who don't, seeing decreases in difficult student behaviors, decreases in negative interactions, and increased compliance among students (Singh et al. 2013). Mindfulness practice can also improve your well-being and reduces stress.

> When educators make time to relax through mindful practices, they give their bodies and minds time to restore and heal from the day-to-day stressors they experience. An activity like taking deep breaths in and out is one example of a tool educators can use to slow down a racing body and mind and bring them back into the present moment. . . . Mindfulness approaches may help build a protective buffer for educators who face many daily stressors in their jobs. (Nicholson et al. 2020, 159)

Your mindfulness practice takes only as much time as you want to devote to it—anywhere from a few minutes to a few hours a day, though most people prefer doing short meditations or breathing exercises. And it costs nothing.

The Foundation for a Mindful Society (2019) suggests the following exercise as a starter for those who are just beginning a mindfulness practice:

1. Set aside some time. You don't need a meditation cushion or bench, or any sort of special equipment to access your mindfulness skills—just time and space.

2. Observe the present moment as it is. The aim of mindfulness is not quieting the mind, or attempting to achieve a state of eternal calm. The goal is to pay attention to the present moment, without judgment.

3. Let your judgments roll by. When you notice judgments arise during your practice, make a mental note of them and let them pass.

4. Return to observing the present moment as it is. Our minds often get carried away in thought. That's why mindfulness is the practice of returning, again and again, to the present moment.

5. Be kind to your wandering mind. Don't judge yourself for whatever thoughts crop up. Just practice recognizing when your mind has wandered off, and gently bring it back.

This Foundation for a Mindful Society provides guidance on many meditations, including a compassion meditation and a guided meditation for easing into sleep (visit www.mindful.org). Look for free mindfulness apps to download to your smartphone or tablet. Many allow you to customize meditations and breathing exercises, and some, like UCLA Mindful, are available in both Spanish and English. Mindfulness has become such a popular tool that it is now considered a mainstream practice.

6. Contemplate nature.

Study after study shows that being in nature reduces stress hormones and improves the immune system (Gleiser 2018). Benefits, including improved memory and attention spans, increased levels of serotonin (the feel-good neurotransmitter), improved performance on tasks requiring sustained focus, and increased energy levels, begin accruing after spending as little as 20 minutes in nature (Biemans 2018; Green 2011).

Shinrin-yoku, or forest bathing, as described in Chapter 6, is particularly restorative. You can enjoy the same documented benefits of forest bathing in something as simple as a walk in a park. Just being outside in nature has positive effects on the brain:

> A walk in the park may soothe the mind and, in the process, change the workings of our brains in ways that improve our mental health. . . . City dwellers have a higher risk for anxiety, depression and other mental illnesses than people living outside urban centers. Various studies have found that urban dwellers with little access to green spaces have a higher incidence of psychological problems than people living near parks and that city dwellers who visit natural environments have lower levels of stress hormones immediately afterward than people who have not recently been outside. (Reynolds 2015)

As more of the population lives in urban areas (Gleiser 2018), deliberately choosing to spend time in nature is more and more needed. In fact, a term has been coined to describe the condition of a disconnection from nature—*psychoterratic* (Livni 2019). Having this condition brings even more stress.

Try to schedule time each day to be in nature. Whether hiking, forest bathing, walking through an arboretum, sitting in a park, throwing pebbles into a creek, or just being outside in the fresh air enjoying the birds, squirrels, and flowers, being outdoors will reduce stress and improve your mood. If you live in an area without easy or safe access to an outdoor area, consider spending time either at the beginning or end of the day or during your scheduled break time in the outdoor area where you take the children in your program to play.

Even looking at nature photos provides benefits (Green 2011). According to Dr. Marc Berman of the Rotman Research Institute in Toronto, staring at nature photos in a quiet room for 10 minutes provides a cognitive boost.

7. Embrace gratitude.

Appreciating what you have received, both tangible and not, helps you focus on what you have—not what you lack (Colker & Koralek 2019). Gratitude is also an excellent way to enhance self-care. "Practicing gratitude on a regular basis has been associated with enhanced optimism, better sleep, fewer physical ailments, and lower levels of anxiety and depression" (van Woerkom 2019).

As van Woerkom notes, numerous research studies have established a link between practicing gratitude and lowering stress and enhancing mental health. In particular, gratitude has been linked to helping individuals overcome trauma and PTSD. Gratitude has the power to reduce toxic emotions such as envy, regret, and resentment and replace them with feelings of satisfaction and happiness. It can decrease aggression, improve self-concept, and make people feel good about themselves. Gratitude can also help you do your job better, as it increases decision-making capabilities, enhances productivity, and increases empathy (L!fe Solutions Counseling 2018).

To include gratitude in your self-care agenda, try some of the following activities:

> Write a thank-you note to someone important in your life, perhaps someone you have never thanked.

> Keep a gratitude journal. Spending just five minutes a day writing down things you are grateful for will increase your long-term well-being by more than 10 percent daily (L!fe Solutions Counseling 2018).

> Count your blessings. Schedule time to sit down each week to reflect on all the good things in your life and think about how they make you feel.

> Practice a gratitude meditation. Doing this just one time can instill feelings of gratitude (Rao & Kemper 2017). You can find a gratitude meditation that suits you online.

8. Do something that will make you feel good about yourself.

Similar to practicing gratitude is being able to feel productive. This can range from going through your closet and throwing out the junk that has accumulated to writing that article you always wanted to and submitting it for publication. Think about your mental to-do list and all those projects you'd like to accomplish but never had time for. Which one can you start today?

Many people feel good about themselves when they reach out to others. Giving back to one's community through volunteer work can bring inner satisfaction. Your first inclination might be to help children or support people experiencing problems. But instead of extending your professional life into volunteer work and risking further compassion fatigue, consider entirely different opportunities such as volunteering at a museum or at a local theatre, cooking meals at a soup kitchen, or running a book drive for your public library.

If you feel strongly about a public issue or want to support a politician or party, these organizations crave volunteers. Lend your talents to letter-writing campaigns, stuffing envelopes, or going door to door on their behalf. Taking action on behalf of your beliefs will make you feel better about yourself and help make your values become a reality.

Another way of feeling good about yourself is to enhance your spirituality. You might do this by attending religious services or doing activities that will enrich your inner self. Spiritual self-care, though difficult to define, involves reflection and introspection on how to best have a life well lived. The Chopra Center (Williams 2019) describes it this way:

> A practice in spiritual self-care quiets the mind and helps to calm the turbulence within, leaving space to begin feeling and honoring what your heart yearns for, and having the courage to take the necessary action for good change. Your body and emotions can't lie; when you are truly happy and thriving you will know it at your core.

9. Put your thoughts down. Try journaling.

Many people find that putting their thoughts down on paper or a computer helps them see things more clearly. This low-cost activity can be done anywhere.

Research has shown that just the act of recording one's thoughts has positive results, particularly for those who have PTSD. It not only helps users find an acceptable way of expressing anger and frustration, but reduces body tension, and restores focus. Nicholson and colleagues (2020) ascribe these benefits to journaling for early childhood educators who use this technique:

> When you translate your experiences into "graspable" language, you free yourself from mentally being tangled in traumas.

> Journaling creates a "pause" button that prevents impulsive reactions.

> It increases empathy for yourself and others.

> It increases self-awareness of sensations, emotions, thoughts, and behaviors.

> Journaling helps you see all of the characters in your story, not just yourself. (151)

Journaling can also help users reflect on their feelings in such a way that they can focus on finding something good in all the negative feelings they are experiencing. This phenomenon is known as *post-traumatic growth*—the ability to find meaning in and have positive life changes following a traumatic event (Tull 2020). Much as the heart of your work with children is healing-centered, post-traumatic growth is your way of triumphing over compassion fatigue.

While there is no right or wrong way to journal—only what works for you—you might search online for suggestions on using journaling to address stress and trauma. For example, check out the article "How Journaling Can Help with PTSD" by Matthew Tull (2020) to identify steps you might employ. Over time, you can go back and look at your entries to see how your thinking and feelings have evolved.

10. Lobby for a hobby.

Your first thought on reading this may be that hobbies are frivolous—indulgences for those with extra time and money to burn. Or you may wonder how with your plate so full you could possibly squeeze in time for a hobby. But hobbies have a lot more to offer than may be apparent at first glance.

In most enthusiasts' minds, "hobbies are a corner of our existence over which we have the impression of control, a sphere in which we feel we can achieve a kind of mastery usually denied to us in our wider personal and professional lives" (Preston 2016).

Hobbies belong in your self-care regimen for several important reasons (Brook 2018, Moments for "Me" 2017; Skilled at Life, n.d.; Singh 2014):

> Hobbies provide an escape from everyday stresses. They let you relax and seek pleasure in activities that aren't associated with work, chores, or other responsibilities.

> Hobbies contribute to psychological well-being. One study found that workers recovered more quickly from the demands of their working lives if they engaged in hobbies in their free time (Eschleman et al. 2014). Likewise, the study found that "the more people engaged in their hobbies, the more likely they were to come up with creative solutions to problems on the job. And no matter what the hobby was, these people were also more likely to go out of their way to help co-workers" (Singh 2014).

> Hobbies provide a sense of purpose in life beyond your work life.

> Hobbies can improve memory (reading or doing crossword puzzles), tap into your creative side (painting, woodworking, or cake decorating), and develop flexibility and physical skills (yoga, hiking, or mountain climbing).

> Hobbies can help your social life and create a bond with others.

> Hobbies build self-efficacy and increase confidence and self-esteem as you take pride in your accomplishments.

> Hobbies provide experiences and stories you can share with others as well as specialized knowledge you can teach to others.

Hobbies don't have to require a lot of money (think reading, running, playing in a band or singing in a chorus, writing poetry) and demand only as much time as you feel comfortable investing.

If you don't currently pursue any hobbies, think about what interests you most—maybe something you enjoyed in childhood, like swimming and playing soccer, or gardening or painting. Or perhaps there's something you've never tried that you always wished you could do, like scrapbooking or learning to play bridge. Give yourself permission to learn how. Putting time in your schedule to follow a passion will reinvigorate you and build your confidence. You'll become a re-energized teacher.

*11. Think positive. Reframe your negative thoughts.

Learning how to reframe pessimistic thoughts is known as cognitive restructuring. Part of cognitive behavioral therapy (CBT), this can be done at home and has been shown to be effective in treating depression and anxiety. The NCTSN (2011) suggests that combining this strategy with mindfulness may be particularly effective in addressing compassion fatigue. We starred this strategy for this reason as one you should consider adding to your self-care regimen.

As noted in Chapter 4, optimism can be learned (Seligman 2005). By going through the ABCDE model outlined in that chapter, where it was presented as being helpful to use with children, you can learn to reframe your own negative thinking (Hall & Pearson 2004).

When you have an experience that triggers pessimistic thoughts, use self-talk to walk your thoughts from A (adverse event) to E (energization) (based on Seligman 2005, 2007):

A = An **adverse** event occurs.

B = You immediately have some negative **beliefs** and thoughts about the adverse event.

C = You experience the **consequences** of having these thoughts and beliefs, including negative emotions.

D = You intentionally **dispute** your pessimistic beliefs.

E = You feel **energized** when you successfully dispute your negative thoughts and realize that the situation is not as you initially believed.

It will take more than one attempt at this process to transform your pessimism into optimism. Practice this exercise every time you start thinking negatively about yourself, your teaching, and your situation. Stress and trauma have a way of making everything seem hopeless. However, if you make a conscious effort to rebut those negative thoughts, you can transform your outlook to one that is hopeful. With time and effort, reframing beliefs, thoughts, and emotions is possible and can become your regular way of thinking.

When you make cognitive restructuring a part of your self-care routine, you will make inroads against the symptoms of compassion fatigue and position yourself to be a role model for children on thinking positively. Learning to think optimistically also has great personal benefits, including better physical and emotional health, longer life, and greater career satisfaction (Colker & Koralek 2019; Seligman 2005). Optimism also leads to greater self-efficacy, problem-solving skill, and the ability to learn from your mistakes (Seligman 2007). If you reframe the negative thinking associated with trauma into positive thoughts, you'll be a happier, more satisfied person.

12. Create or join a peer group.

Peer support groups are effective for managing "the weight of trauma" (Lander 2018). In the same way you might meet with colleagues to form curriculum committees, plan professional development events, and confer on the best approaches for individual children and families, you can formally band together to address mental health needs. Though it takes effort and coordination, you'll all benefit from supporting each other. Here are some suggestions for getting started:

> Establish a regular meeting time, perhaps weekly, biweekly, or monthly. Let your supervisor know of your plans and ask whether they can facilitate the group's operation.

> Find a meeting space where you will be undisturbed.

> Become familiar with the triggers and symptoms of secondary stress so you know what to watch for in yourself and your colleagues.

> Arrange to have a mental health professional either in attendance or on standby for support, if possible.

> Focus the sessions as check-ins with each other as to how you feel and how your colleagues think you are faring.

> Actively find ways to support each other in self-care. You might wish to join each other for some fun out-of-school activities where you make talking about work off limits.

> Revisit your progress from meeting to meeting, deciding which approaches work best for everyone.

> Be available for mutual support between scheduled meeting times.

13. Request reflective supervision.

Practicing TIC requires reflection. If you are part of a school or program in which you are supervised and the program does not already provide reflective supervision, advocate for access to this important support.

Reflective supervision, much like reflective teaching, involves active listening and thoughtful questioning by both educators and their supervisors. This technique has been used effectively with educators who are experiencing the effects of secondary trauma. The organization Zero to Three (2016) describes the practice this way:

> Reflective supervision is not therapy. It is focused on experiences, thoughts, and feelings directly connected with the work. . . . The role of the supervisor is to help the supervisee to answer her own questions and to provide the support and knowledge necessary to guide decision-making. In addition, the supervisor provides an empathetic, nonjudgmental ear to the supervisee. Working through complex emotions in a "safe place" allows the supervisee to manage the stress she experiences on the job. It also allows the staff person to experience the very sort of relationship that she is expected to provide for [children] and families.

To work as intended, the process needs to be fully collaborative and ongoing. With the emphasis on reflection, educators have an opportunity to determine how they think they are doing—both what's working well and where they could use some support. Both educators and supervisors weigh in on how trauma is affecting educators and what other types of self-care might be warranted. Reflective supervision thus builds teamwork, respect, and stability while enhancing mental health.

14. Seek support when you need it.

Just better tending to your basic needs and adding some balance to your life may be all you need to feel re-energized. However, if you feel angry all the time, want to run away, or feel you cannot go on any longer, a licensed mental health professional can help you develop an appropriate strategy for moving forward. It is critical to get professional help if you feel like you are unable to function or perform the basic activities of daily living—including your job. Even if you are not at a crisis point, getting professional help can help you sort through what is happening.

Always remember that there is absolutely no shame in seeking help. It is a sign of strength rather than weakness to recognize that counseling can help you better process the stories and voices of trauma you deal with daily.

*15. Take action. Make a self-care plan.

Once you are aware of the many self-care techniques you might try, the next step is to develop an action plan. This activity has been starred because you need a self-care plan to help you make these activities a part of your daily routine. By mapping out a plan for implementing the activities you want to focus on, you will have a blueprint for making self-care a part of your life.

Ask yourself some reflective questions:

> How do I cope with stress now?

> What do I do for self-care now?

> How is my current self-care program (if you have one) working for me?

> What do I like that I am doing and plan to continue?

> What do I dislike? Are there things I am doing now that I'm likely to quit in the future?

> How do my current self-care activities relate to the list of strategies presented above? Is there overlap?

> Assuming that I will work on strategies 1, 5, and 11 first, which other ones do I think are most important *and* ones that I might do?

> Are there some activities that I will never do that I should cross off this list right now?

> What are my top choices from the remaining 11 strategies?

> What factors would help me make my top strategies an ongoing part of my lifestyle?

The next step is to turn the strategies you want to try into goals you can realistically accomplish. While you will eventually want to make goals for the three suggested activities (1, 5, and 11) in addition to your other top choices, we suggest that you begin slowly—with only two or three goals to start. This will keep you from feeling overwhelmed and allow you to adjust as needed. After you have incorporated these first few goals into your routine and are seeing benefits from doing them, add another goal or two.

In formulating your self-care goals, we suggest using an approach developed in 1981 in the management field—SMART goals (Doran 1981). SMART goals are expressed in a way that is clearly articulated and can be readily assessed. This is because they are

> Specific

> Measurable

> Assignable

> Realistic

> Time related

Here's how this might work. Suppose you want to develop goals for these three strategies you have selected to begin your self-care regimen:

Strategy 1: Be kind to yourself

Strategy 5: Cultivate mindfulness

Strategy 9: Try journaling

Now look at each strategy one at a time, beginning with Strategy 1. While you might ultimately have several SMART goals under Strategy 1 related to such things as nutrition, sleep, exercise, spending more time with friends, or going to church more regularly, let's assume for the purpose of this exercise that you feel pretty good about most of these areas, but you know you could use more exercise and need to get outside more often for some fresh air. Your knee's not in great shape, but you still like to take walks, and you think you might be able to convince your partner to accompany you—at least some of the time.

With these considerations in mind, you can formulate a SMART goal by thinking about these SMART-related questions (Haughey 2014; MindTools, n.d.):

> Specific: What exactly are you trying to accomplish? Why is this goal important to you? What resources or limits are involved?

> Measurable: How much effort will it take? How many people are involved? How will you know you accomplished it?

> Assignable: Who will do it?

> Realistic: Is this worthwhile? What results can realistically be achieved given available resources?

> Time related: When specifically can it be achieved? What can I do today?

Based on the considerations already mentioned, a SMART goal for Strategy 1 might be "I will take a 30-minute walk on Saturdays and Sundays."

For Strategy 5, you might come up with "Each night I will meditate for five minutes before I go to bed."

A SMART goal for Strategy 9 could be "Three times a week, I will spend 15–20 minutes writing down my thoughts about how I feel at the end of my workday on my smartphone."

Once you have your goals written down, display them on your refrigerator or post them on a bulletin board in your home. We suggest that you also keep track of them more formally by using a weekly chart to track your progress. Having a chart will allow you to assess your ability to incorporate these goals into your daily life— which is the point of having measurable goals. Review your progress at the end of each week and suggest modifications for the coming week. Once you get into a flow that works for you, you may need to use the chart only to record and monitor your use of the self-care goals and strategies.

By taking a proactive approach to self-care, you can ensure that you are teaching at the top of your game. Feeling confident and assured, you can work with children and families to achieve post-traumatic growth.

A Path Forward

With your healing-centered interventions, perseverance, and compassionate teaching, the effects of trauma can be turned around—for the children you teach, their families, and you. Children's histories do not have to be the prologue to the rest of their lives. As trauma therapist and author Karen Saakvitne proclaims, "Everyone has a right to have a present and future that are not completely dominated and dictated by the past" (Klinic Community Health Centre 2013, 4). You can be the change agent who gives children that opportunity to rewrite their life story with promise and hope.

APPENDIX One

Resources for Educators

Print Resources

Culturally Responsive Self-Care Practices for Early Childhood Educators, by Julie Nicholson, Priya Shimpi Driscoll, Julie Kurtz, Doménica Márquez, and Lawanda Wesley. 2020. Routledge.

The Deepest Well: Healing the Long-Term Effects of Childhood Adversity, by Nadine Burke Harris. 2018. Houghton Mifflin Harcourt.

Fostering Resilient Learners: Strategies for Creating a Trauma-Sensitive Classroom, by Kristin Souers, with Pete Hall. 2016. ASCD.

High-Quality Early Childhood Programs: The What, Why, and How, by Laura J. Colker and Derry Koralek. 2018. Redleaf Press.

Reaching and Teaching Children Exposed to Trauma, by Barbara Sorrels. 2015. Gryphon House.

Reaching and Teaching Children Who Hurt: Strategies for Your Classroom, by Susan E. Craig. 2008. Brookes Publishing.

Teaching to Strengths: Supporting Students Living with Trauma, Violence, and Chronic Stress, by Debbie Zacarian, Lourdes Alvarez-Ortiz, and Judie Haynes. 2017. ASCD.

Trauma-Informed Practices for Early Childhood Educators: Relationship-Based Approaches that Support Healing and Build Resilience in Young Children, by Julie Nicholson, Linda Perez, and Julie Kurtz. 2019. Routledge.

Trauma-Sensitive Mindfulness: Practices for Safe and Transformative Healing, by David T. Treleaven. 2108. W.W. Norton & Co.

Digital Resources

Asking the Question that Counts: Educators and Early Childhood Trauma, by The Council for Professional Recognition. www.cdacouncil.org /storage/documents/Media_Room/Asking_the _Question_that_Counts_Final.pdf

Child Development and Trauma Guide, by the Department of Human Services, State of Victoria, Australia. www.dcp.wa.gov.au/ChildProtection /ChildAbuseAndNeglect/Documents /ChildDevelopmentAndTraumaGuide.pdf

Child Trauma Toolkit for Educators, by The National Child Traumatic Stress Network. www.nctsn.org /resources/child-trauma-toolkit-educators

Creating Trauma Sensitive Classrooms, by Katie Statman-Weil. www.naeyc.org/resources/pubs/yc /may2015/trauma-sensitive-classrooms

The Heart of Learning and Teaching: Compassion, Resiliency, and Academic Success, by Ray Wolpow, Mona M. Johnson, Ron Hertel, and Susan O. Kincaid. www.k12.wa.us/student-success/health-safety /mental-social-behavioral-health/compassionate -schools-learning-and-1

Helping Traumatized Children Learn, by Susan F. Cole, Jessica Greenwald O'Brien, M. Geron Gadd, Joel Ristuccia, D. Luray Wallace, and Michael Gregory. https://traumasensitiveschools.org/tlpi-publications /download-a-free-copy-of-helping-traumatized -children-learn

How Schools Can Help Students Recover from Traumatic Experiences: A Tool Kit for Supporting Long-Term Recovery, by Lisa H. Jaycox, Lindsey K. Morse, Terri Tanielian, and Bradley D. Stein. www .rand.org/content/dam/rand/pubs/technical _reports/2006/RAND_TR413.pdf

Traumatic Experiences, from Sesame Street in Communities. www.sesamestreetincommunities.org /topics/traumatic-experiences

Trauma-Informed The Trauma Toolkit, 2nd edition, by Klinic Community Health Centre. http://trauma -informed.ca/wp-content/uploads/2013/10/Trauma -informed_Toolkit.pdf

Trauma Toolkit: Tools to Support the Learning and Development of Students Experiencing Childhood and Adolescent Trauma, by First Book in partnership with Maryland State Education Association. http:// taaaconline.org/wp-content/uploads/2018/03 /Trauma-Toolkit-for-Educators.pdf

Violence in the Lives of Children, by NAEYC. Position statement. https://naeyc.org/sites/default/files /globally-shared/downloads/PDFs/resources /position-statements/PSVIOL98.PDF

Wisconsin's Trauma-Sensitive Schools Online Professional Development. https://dpi.wi.gov/sspw /mental-health/trauma

Video Clips and Webinars

Broken Places. Roger Weisberg. 55-minute film on resilience in children. https://www.pbs.org/show /broken-places

Effective Strategies in Addressing Trauma in Children of Incarcerated Parents, SAMHSA. 1½ -hour webinar. www.youtube.com/watch?v=YdhI -AoHkuw

Trauma, Brain and Relationship: Helping Children Heal. Dr. Bruce Perry and other experts on early childhood trauma. 5½-minute video. www.youtube .com/watch?v=RYj7YYHmbQs

Trauma-Sensitive Classrooms. Barbara Sorrels and Katie Statman-Weil. 57-minute webinar. www.youtube.com/watch?v=mjG3xNxtU1E

Understanding How an Immigrant Family Navigates Family Trauma, NCTSN. 1½-hour webinar. www.nctsn.org/resources/understanding-how-an-immigrant-family-navigates-family-trauma

Understanding Trauma and Promoting Resilience in Vulnerable Children, SAMHSA. 67-minute webinar. www.youtube.com/watch?v=CyrfoqKFiOo

Web Resources

CASEL (Collaborative for Academic, Social, and Emotional Learning). Provides resources on evidence-based social and emotional learning for preschool through high school. www.casel.org

CDC (The Centers for Disease Control and Prevention). Houses and distributes multiple reports, training modules, and handbooks related to childhood trauma. www.cdc.gov

Center for the Developing Child at Harvard University. Provides science-based research and innovation outcomes to benefit children facing adversity. Develops and disseminates print, audio, and video materials on trauma. www.developingchild.harvard.edu

CTC (Center for Trauma and the Community). Provides culturally sensitive innovative materials for low-income users free of charge. www.ctc.georgetown.edu

NAEYC (National Association for the Education of Young Children). Publishes numerous articles related to trauma and resilience. NAEYC.org

National Center for PTSD, US Department of Veterans Affairs. Information and tools about PTSD from the world's leading research and educational center of excellence on PTSD and traumatic stress. www.ptsd.va.gov

NCPMI (National Center for Pyramid Model Innovations). Brings together research scholars who have developed the Pyramid Model for Promoting Social and Emotional Competence in Infants and Young Children. www.challengingbehavior.cbcs.usf.edu

NCTSN (The National Child Traumatic Stress Network). National resource for developing and disseminating evidence-based interventions, trauma-informed services, and public and professional education. www.nctsn.org

SAMHSA (Substance Abuse and Mental Health Services Administration). Addresses the impact of trauma on individuals, families, and communities as a behavioral health concern. www.samhsa.gov

Teaching Tolerance. Provides free resources to teachers, administrators, counselors, and other practitioners who work with children from kindergarten through high school. www.tolerance.org

Zero to Three. Develops training materials, research reports, and videos on trauma-informed practice for infants and toddlers. www.zerotothree.org

APPENDIX TWO

Picture Books About Trauma

Abuse and Neglect

Clover's Secret, by Christine M. Winn. 1996. Fairview Press.

The Day My Daddy Lost His Temper: Empowering Kids That Have Witnessed Domestic Violence, by Dr. Carol Santana McCleary. 2014. CreateSpace Independent Publishing Platform.

Fawn's Touching Tale: A Story for Children Who Have Been Sexually Abused, by Agnes Wohl and Irene Wineman Marcus. 2018. Stress Free Press.

Mommy's Black Eye, by William George Bentrim. 2009. CreateSpace Independent Publishing Platform.

No More Secrets for Me: Sexual Abuse Is A Secret No Child Should Have to Keep, by Oralee Wachter. 2002. Little, Brown and Co.

A Place for Starr. Children and Their Experience of Family Violence: A Story of Hope, by Howard Schor. 2017. CreateSpace Independent Publishing Platform.

Somebody Cares: A Guide for Kids Who Have Experienced Neglect, by Susan Farber Straus. 2016. Magination Press. Also available in Chinese.

Addiction

Addie's Mom Isn't Home Anymore, by Genia Calvin. 2019. Independently published.

Hey, Kiddo: How I Lost My Mother, Found My Father, and Dealt with Family Addiction, by Jarrett J. Krosoczka. 2018. Graphix.

When A Family Is In Trouble: Children Can Cope With Grief From Drug and Alcohol Addiction, by Marge Heedaard. 1996. Woodland Press.

Wylie's Wishes: Andy's Story (A Child's Journey Through Trauma), by Wylie. 2019. Independently published.

Coping With Scary Experiences and Feelings

Alex and the Scary Things: A Story to Help Children Who have Experienced Something Scary, by Melissa Moses. 2015. Jessica Kingsley Publishers.

Bear Feels Scared, by Karma Wilson. 2011. Little Simon.

Bomji and Spotty's Frightening Adventure: A Story About How to Recover from a Scary Experience, by Anne Westcott and C.C. Alicia Hu. 2017. Jessica Kingsley Publishers.

A Flicker of Hope, by Julia Cook. 2018. National Center for Youth Issues.

Good Answers to Tough Questions: Trauma, by Joy Berry. 2010. Joy Berry Books.

Healing Days: A Guide for Kids Who Have Experienced Trauma, by Susan Farber Strauss. 2013. Magination Press.

How Little Coyote Found His Secret Strength: A Story About How to Get Through Hard Times, by Anne Westcott and C.C. Alicia Hu. 2017. Jessica Kingsley Publishers.

I'm Not Scared . . . I'm Prepared, by Julia Cook. 2014. National Center for Youth Services.

Jenny Is Scared: When Sad Things Happen In The World, by Carol Shuman. 2003. Magination Press.

Letting Go of Yucky Feelings or Drop the Lemons, by Asaf Shani. 2018. Independently published.

My Breath Loves Me, by Claire E. Hallinan. 2019. Self-published.

Once I Was Very Scared, by Chandra Ghosh Ippen. *Una Vez Tuve Mucho Mucho Miedo,* Spanish edition. 2017. Piplo Productions.

The Stormy Secret, by Jed Jurchenko. 2019. Independently published.

Trauma: Teaching Kids All About Trauma, by Robert D. Edelman. 2015. CreateSpace Independent Publishing Platform.

Whimsy's Heavy Things, by Julie Kraulis. 2013. Tundra Books.

Death

Always and Forever, by Alan Durant. 2013. Random House Children's Publishers.

The Goodbye Book, by Todd Parr. 2015. Little, Brown Books for Young Readers.

I Remember Miss Perry, by Pat Brisson. 2006. Dial Publishers.

The Scar, by Charlotte Moundlic. 2011. Candlewick Press.

Tear Soup: A Recipe for Healing After Loss, by Pat Schwiebert and Chuck DeKlyen. 2005. Grief Watch.

Where Did My Friend Go? Helping Children Cope With a Traumatic Death, by Azamira H. Maker. 2017. Aspiring Families Press.

Family Separation/Divorce

Countdown 'Til Daddy Comes Home, by Kristin Ayyar. 2013. Mascot Books.

Daddy's Boots, by Sandra Miller Linhart. 2017. Lionhart Group Project.

Family Changes: Explaining Divorce to Children, by Azmaira H. Maker. 2015. Aspiring Families Press.

How Sprinkle the Pig Escaped the River of Tears: A Story About Being Apart From Loved Ones, by Anne Westcott and C.C. Alicia Hu. 2017. Jessica Kingsley Publishers.

You Weren't With Me, by Chandra Ghosh Ippen. 2019. *Cuando No Estabas Conmigo,* Spanish edition. 2019. Piplo Productions.

Foster Care/Adoption

Families Change: A Book For Children Experiencing Termination of Parental Rights, by Julie Nelson. 2006. Free Spirit Press.

Henry and Grammy Kay Talk About Adoption, by Cindy K. Clark. 2019. Independently published.

Kids Need to Be Safe: A Book for Children in Foster Care, by Julie Nelson. 2005. Free Spirit Press.

Maybe Days: A Book for Children in Foster Care, by Jennifer Wilgocki. 2002. American Psychological Association.

Murphy's Three Homes: A Story for Children in Foster Care, by Jan Levinson Gilman. 2008. Magination Press.

Speranza's Sweater: A Child's Journey Through Foster Care and Adoption, by Marcy Pusey. 2018. Miramare Ponte Press.

Homelessness

I May Not Have A Home: A Children's Book About Homelessness and Dignity, by Andrea Landriault. 2017. CreateSpace Independent Publishing Platform.

A Place to Stay: A Shelter Story, by Erin Gunti. 2019. Barefoot Books.

A Shelter in Our Car, by Monica Gunning. 2013. Lee and Low Books.

Still A Family: A Story About Homelessness, by Brenda Reeves Sturgis. 2017. Albert Whitman.

Illness/Hospitalization

Mommy Has To Stay In Bed, by Annette Rivlin-Gutman. 2009. BookSurge Publishing.

The Playdate Kids: Dakota's Mom Goes to the Hospital, by Annie Thiel. 2007. Playdate Publishing.

When Pete's Dad Got Sick: A Book About Chronic Illness, by Kathleen Long Bostrom. 2004. Zonderkidz.

Why Does Mommy Hurt? Helping Children Cope with the Challenges of Having a Caregiver with Chronic Pain, Fibromyalgia, or Autoimmune Disease, by Elizabeth M. Christy. 2015. Outskirts Press.

Incarceration

My Daddy's in Jail, by Anthony Corcio. 2015. ICG Children's.

The Night Dad Went to Jail, by Melissa Higgins. 2014. Picture Window Books.

Visiting Day, by Jaqueline Woodson. 2015. Puffin Books.

When Daronte's Father Went to Prison, by Kimberly Ballou. 2017. CreateSpace Independent Publishing Platform.

Natural Disasters

Earthquakes! An Earthshattering Book on the Science of Plate Tectonics, Earth Science for Kids. Prodigy Wizard Books. 2016.

Elmer and the Flood, by David McKee. 2015. Andersen Press.

Hurricanes! by Gail Gibbons. 2009. Hurricane House.

River Friendly, River Wild, by Jane Kurtz. 2000. Simon & Schuster Books for Young Readers.

Tornadoes! by Gail Gibbons. 2009. Holiday House.

When the Ground Shakes, by Irit Almog and Shoshana Wheeler. 2018. Children 911 Resources.

Violence

Latoya's Downtown Day, by Patricia Moore. 2018. Independently published.

Stan the Timid Turtle: Helping Children Cope With Fears About School Violence, by Laura Fox. 2014. New Horizon Press.

A Terrible Thing Happened: A Story for Children Who Have Witnessed Violence or Trauma, by Margaret M. Holmes. 2000. Magination Press.

Why Did It Happen? Helping Children Cope In A Violent World, by Janice Cohn 1994. William Morrow & Co.

It is important that you help families support their children when they have experienced trauma. Here are three handouts you can photocopy and send home with families.

What Is Trauma in Children?

Dear Families,

Trauma is a scary, dangerous, or violent event that a child experiences or witnesses that overwhelms their ability to cope. Each child will interpret and respond to trauma differently. Something that is very difficult for one child may not bother another child. Here are ways a child might experience and react to trauma along with some things you can do to help your child.

Sources of Trauma

Trauma can come from different sources and aspects of a child's life. These can include

> Abuse or neglect
> Separation from family or trusted caregivers
> Violence in their home or community
> A serious car crash or other harmful incident
> A natural disaster
> Substance abuse in their home
> Death of someone important to the child

How Children React to Trauma

A child may show signs like

> Reliving the traumatic event
> Having nightmares
> Being irritable or hyperalert
> Having trouble sleeping
> Having negative thoughts about themselves
> Isolating themselves or seeming detached
> Being extra clingy to trusted adults
> Reverting to behaviors they have outgrown
> Acting out the trauma through their play

What You Can Do

> Ask yourself, "Did something happen in my child's life that caused harm or made them feel threatened?" Remember that each child is unique. Also, as an adult you will look at things differently than your child does.
> Learn more about possible reactions to trauma and what it can look like in children. Two great resources are the National Child Traumatic Stress Network (www.nctsn.org) and Child Mind Institute (https://childmind.org/topics/concerns/trauma-and-grief).
> Help your child feel safe. Be there for your child and remind them of all the ways that their family and their teacher are there to help them.
> Reassure your child that they aren't responsible for the trauma. Many children worry that it is their fault something happened.
> Allow your child to express their fears out loud and through their play and art.
> Be patient with your child. Working through trauma happens on their own time and in their own way. If you see behavior changes, remember that it is not because your child is trying to be difficult.
> If these reactions or symptoms persist for more than a few weeks, talk to a mental health provider. Your pediatrician, early childhood program, spiritual leader, or community organizations can help you find one that meets the needs of your child and your family.

Dealing with Challenging Behaviors Caused by Trauma

Dear Families,

If your child has experienced a traumatic event, you might see some of the following behaviors. Try some of the tips to help your child feel safe and able to manage their fears.

If your child is acting like this . . .	Try doing this . . .
Being fearful, clinging, and unusually scared of being left alone or separated from you	Offer frequent reassurances: "I will be here to pick you up after school—just like I do every day." Remind your child that there are photos of family members at the program that they can look at if they feel lonely. Record yourself reading your child's favorite book that your child can listen to at the program. Create rituals for when you drop off and pick up your child: sing a song together or make up a special greeting. Make and post a picture schedule at home to show when you will drop them off at school and pick them up and what you will do after school.
Expressing fears that the traumatic incident isn't over or will return	Provide calm, honest explanations as often as necessary. For example, if your child has experienced a hurricane or wildfires: "People are working hard to get everything back to normal." "We are safe from the flood. The waters are gone." "If you get scared, come hold my hand and we'll talk about it." "This rain is just regular rain. It won't turn into a hurricane." "The smoke in the sky is from a factory chimney. There are no wildfires."
Regressing to behaviors the child has outgrown, such as thumb sucking, wetting their pants, or using baby talk	Remain calm. Have a matter-of-fact conversation about the behavior. Take care not to make a big deal of it, and don't criticize or shame your child. As your child recovers and feels more confident, the behaviors will disappear.
Sleeping fitfully, not being able to fall asleep, having nightmares or screaming during sleep	Spend extra time with your child before bedtime or napping. Stay close and perhaps rub your child's back or belly. Play calming music and encourage your child to pick a favorite stuffed animal to sleep with. Reassure your child with fact-based explanations: "The monsters in dreams are caused by our thoughts. They aren't real."
Re-creating the trauma in their play	Join your child's play and ask open-ended questions to find what your child thinks is happening. Provide ways for your child to feel some control over the traumatic incident: "What could you do to make your doll feel safe?" "Where could the people go if they have no home to live in?"
Acting out; aggressively hitting or kicking others	Let the child know that while it's okay to be angry, it's not okay to hurt anyone else: "Everyone gets angry at times. If you feel like hitting, you can talk to me and we can figure out how to get the angry feelings out of you in a safe way. I cannot let you hit anyone, though."
Acting withdrawn; not talking	Provide extra attention. Let the child know that you are there for them if they want to talk, but don't force them to. Suggest painting or drawing or pounding clay. Read books to the child, offering comments like "The turtle in the story is very kind. There were a lot of caring people helping out when your daddy had to leave, too."

Adapted from L.J. Colker, "Being a Helper: Helping Children to Feel Safe and Secure Following Disasters," *Teaching Young Children* 11 (February/March 2018), 17–20. www.naeyc.org/resources/pubs/tyc/feb2018/being-helper-supporting-children-feel-safe-and-secure -after-disasters.

Creating and Using a Glitter Jar

Dear Families,

This activity helps children understand what their brain looks like when they are worried, upset, or thinking about something they cannot control. By watching the glitter settle in the jar from its flurried state, children can compare it to the way their brain calms down when they are able to regulate their emotions.

1. Begin by making a glitter jar with your child. To do this, you will need a pint or quart-sized canning jar (also known as a Mason jar), distilled water, glitter, vegetable oil, and glycerine. If you search online for "how to make a glitter jar with vegetable oil," you'll find a video to walk you through the steps. Or, you can use water, baking soda, hair gel, and glitter instead. You can also purchase a ready-made glitter jar online or use a snow globe, if you prefer.

2. Tell your child that the glitter jar is like their brain. Ask them to vigorously shake their finished jar. What do they see? They can think of all the glitter falling about as what happens in their brain when their thoughts and emotions feel out of control. Do they think they could use their brain to learn when they are like this?

3. Ask your child to put the jar down. Together discuss what they see as the glitter settles down. Take some deep breaths together. Have your child put their hands on their tummy. Can they feel how their breathing is calming down like the glitter?

4. Now look through the jar. Can they see the other side? Did the glitter go away? No, it's just settled down. That's like the upsetting thoughts and feelings in our brains. They don't disappear, they just settle down when we do some breathing and let our thoughts and feelings settle. Now we can think clearly again.

Whenever your child is overcome by emotions, try reminding them of this activity with the phrase, "Let's settle our glitter."

Adapted from S.K. Greenland, "Seeing Clearly," Susan K. Greenland blog (May 7, 2017). www.susankaisergreenland.com/listen-1/2017/5/7/seeing-clearly?rq=shake%20the%20ball.

References

ACF (Administration for Children & Families). n.d. a. "Secondary Traumatic Stress. What Is Secondary Traumatic Stress?" *Resource Guide to Trauma-Informed Human Services.* Accessed September 10, 2019. www.acf.hhs.gov/trauma-toolkit/secondary-traumatic-stress.

ACF. n.d. b. "What Is Historical Trauma?" *Resource Guide to Trauma-Informed Human Services.* Accessed January 22, 2020. www.acf.hhs.gov/trauma-toolkit/trauma-concept.

Alber, R. 2018. "When Teachers Experience Empathic Distress." *Edutopia,* April 18. www.edutopia.org/article/when-teachers-experience-empathic-distress.

ALMA (Astrid Lindgren Memorial Award). n.d. "Philip Pullman." Accessed November 3, 2019. http://alma.se/en/About-the-award/ALMA-10-years/Philip-Pullman.

American Counseling Association. 2011. "Vicarious Trauma." Fact Sheet #9. October 10. www.counseling.org/docs/trauma-disaster/fact-sheet-9—vicarious-trauma.pdf.

APA (American Psychological Association). n.d. "Undocumented Americans: What Is It Like to Grow Up as an Undocumented Youth in America?" Accessed October 15, 2019. www.apa.org/topics/immigration/undocumented-video.

Association for Psychological Science. 2014. "Heavily Decorated Classrooms Disrupt Attention and Learning in Young Children." May 27. www.psychologicalscience.org/news/releases/heavily-decorated-classrooms-disrupt-attention-and-learning-in-young-children.html?fbclid=IwAR2a5eKMzBVov1NCTRT1awuDbr3cPGyJvFsrnFZ1t6Y5TUApkb1lFh3_hzM#.XSjivm6rTrc.facebook.

Austin, L.J.E., B. Edwards, R. Chávez, & M. Whitebook. 2019. "Racial Wage Gaps in Early Education Employment." Center for the Study of Child Care Employment, December 19. https://cscce.berkeley.edu/racial-wage-gaps-in-early-education-employment.

Baker, M. 2007. "Music Moves Brain to Pay Attention, Organize Events." *Stanford News,* August 8. https://news.stanford.edu/news/2007/august8/med-music-080807.html.

Becker, B.D., K.C. Gallagher, & R.C. Whitaker. 2017. "Teachers' Dispositional Mindfulness and the Quality of Their Relationships with Children in Head Start Classrooms." *Journal of School Psychology* 65: 40–53. http://isiarticles.com/bundles/Article/pre/pdf/119781.pdf.

Beloglovsky, M., & M. Grant-Groves. 2019. "Promoting Equity Through Play." *Exchange* 41 (3): 57–61.

Berger, T. 2018. "An Inside Look at Trauma-Informed Practices." *Edutopia,* February 5. www.edutopia.org/article/inside-look-trauma-informed-practices.

Bergstrom, C. 2015. "Mindfulness: What It Is and How to Explain It to Kids and Adults." *Blissful Kids,* September 28. https://blissfulkids.com/what-is-mindfulness-and-how-to-explain-it-to-kids.

Berinato, S. 2020. "That Discomfort You're Feeling Is Grief." *Harvard Business Review,* March 23. https://hbr.org/2020/03/that-discomfort-youre-feeling-is-grief.

Biemans, R. 2018. "Self Care: Connecting with Nature." Maryland Coalition of Families, September 13. www.mdcoalition.org/blog/self-care-connecting-with-nature.

Biermeier, M.A. 2015. "Inspired by Reggio Emilia: Emergent Curriculum in Relationship-Driven Learning Environments." *Young Children* 70 (5): 72–79. www.naeyc.org/resources/pubs/yc/nov2015/emergent-curriculum.

Biswas-Diener, R., T.B. Kashdan, & M. Gurpal. 2011. "A Dynamic Approach to Psychological Strength Development and Intervention." *Journal of Positive Psychology* 6 (2): 106–18.

Blair, C., & C.C. Raver. 2016. "Poverty, Stress, and Brain Development: New Directions for Prevention and Intervention." *Academic Pediatrics* 16 (3): S30–S36.

Bride, B. E., M. Radey, & C.R. Figley. 2007. "Measuring Compassion Fatigue." *Clinical Social Work Journal* 35 (3): 155–63.

Brook, J. 2018. "10 Hobbies to Build Confidence and Self-Esteem in Yourself." *Everyday Power,* February 23. https://everydaypower.com/10-hobbies-build -confidence-self-esteem.

Carter, R.T. 2006. "Race-Based Traumatic Stress." *Psychiatric Times* 23 (14). www.psychiatrictimes.com /cultural-psychiatry/race-based-traumatic-stress.

Caspi, Y., B. Ghafoori, S. Smith, & A. Contractor. 2013. "On the Importance of Considering Culture in Defining Trauma." September 24. https://istss.org/public -resources/trauma-blog/2013-october/on-the -importance-of-considering-culture-when-defi.

CDC (Centers for Disease Control and Prevention). 2015. "Fatal Injury Reports, National and Regional, 1999–2015." June 24. https://webappa.cdc.gov/sasweb /ncipc/mortrate10_us.html.

CDC. 2019. "Helping Children with Disabilities Cope with Disaster and Traumatic Events." September 18. www.cdc .gov/ncbddd/disabilityandsafety/trauma.html.

Center on the Developing Child (Center on the Developing Child, Harvard University). n.d. a. "ACEs and Toxic Stress: Frequently Asked Questions." Accessed June 11, 2018. https://developingchild.harvard.edu /resources/aces-and-toxic-stress-frequently-asked -questions.

Center on the Developing Child. n.d. b. "Brain Architecture." Accessed March 14, 2019. https:// developingchild.harvard.edu/science/key-concepts /brain-architecture.

Center on the Developing Child. n.d. c. "Resilience." Accessed July 29, 2018. https://developingchild.harvard .edu/science/key-concepts/resilience.

Center on the Developing Child. n.d. d. "Serve and Return." Accessed July 31, 2018. https://developingchild.harvard .edu/science/key-concepts/serve-and-return.

Center on the Developing Child. n.d. e. "Toxic Stress." Accessed June 11, 2018. https://developingchild.harvard .edu/science/key-concepts/toxic-stress.

Chatterjee, R., & R. Davis. 2017. "How Racism May Cause Black Mothers to Suffer the Death of Their Infants." *NPR Morning Edition*, December 20. www.npr.org/sections /health-shots/2017/12/20/570777510/how-racism-may -cause-black-mothers-to-suffer-the-death-of-their-infants.

Child Mind Institute. n.d. "Kids Who Need a Little Help to Make Friends: What Parents Can Do When Kids Struggle with Social Skills." Accessed August 4, 2019. https:// childmind.org/article/kids-who-need-a-little-help-to -make-friends.

Child Trends. 2016. "Key Facts About Children's Exposure to Violence." Accessed July 18, 2019. www.childtrends .org/indicators/childrens-exposure-to-violence.

Child Trends. 2019. "Adverse Childhood Experiences." March 7. www.childtrends.org/indicators/adverse -experiences.

Children's Bureau (Children's Bureau, Administration for Children & Families). 2016. "Child Maltreatment 2014." January 25. www.acf.hhs.gov/cb/resource/child -maltreatment-2014.

Children's Defense Fund. 2019. "Child Poverty." www.childrensdefense.org/policy/policy-priorities/child -poverty.

Christian, M.D., & O.A. Barbarin. 2001. "Cultural Resources and Psychological Adjustment of African American Children: Effects of Spirituality and Racial Attribution." *Journal of Black Psychology* (27) 1: 43–63.

Clauss-Ehlers, C.S. 2004. "Re-inventing Resilience: A Model of Culturally-Focused Resilient Adaptation." In *Community Planning to Foster Resilience in Children*, eds. C.S. Clauss-Ehlers & M.D. Weist, 27–41. New York: Kluwer Academic Publishers.

Cole, S., A. Eisner, M. Gregory, & J. Ristuccia. 2013. *Creating and Advocating for Trauma-Sensitive Schools.* Helping Traumatized Children Learn 2. Trauma and Learning Policy Initiative. https:// traumasensitiveschools.org/tlpi-publications.

Cole, S.F., J.G. O'Brien, M.G. Gadd, J. Ristuccia, D.L. Wallace, & M. Gregory. 2005. *Helping Traumatized Children Learn: Supportive School Environments for Children Traumatized by Family Violence*. A Report and Policy Agenda. Massachusetts Advocates for Children, Trauma and Learning Policy Initiative. https://traumasensitiveschools.org/wp-content/uploads/2013/06/Helping-Traumatized-Children-Learn.pdf.

Colker, L.J., & D. Koralek. 2018. *High-Quality Early Childhood Programs: The What, Why, and How*. St. Paul, MN: Redleaf.

Colker, L.J., & D. Koralek. 2019. *Making Lemonade: Teaching Young Children to Think Optimistically*. St. Paul, MN: Redleaf.

Collin-Vézina, D., I. Daigneault, & M. Hébert. 2013. "Lessons Learned from Child Sexual Abuse Research: Prevalence, Outcomes, and Preventive Strategies." *Child and Adolescent Psychiatry and Mental Health* 7: 22. www.ncbi.nlm.nih.gov/pmc/articles/PMC3720272.

Collins, K., K. Connors, S. Davis, A. Donohue, S. Gardner, E. Goldblatt, A. Hayward, L. Kiser, F. Strieder, & E. Thompson. 2010. *Understanding the Impact of Trauma and Urban Poverty on Family Systems: Risks, Resilience, and Interventions*. Baltimore, MD: Family Informed Trauma Treatment Center. https://storage.googleapis.com/quantumunitsed-com/materials/1431_0221_Trauma-Urban_Poverty.pdf.

Comas-Díaz, L., G.N. Hall, & H.A. Neville. 2019. "Racial Trauma: Theory, Research, and Healing: Introduction to the Special Issue." *American Psychologist* 74 (1): 1–5. http://dx.doi.org/10.1037/amp0000442.

Compassion Fatigue Awareness Project. n.d. "Recognizing Compassion Fatigue." Accessed August 12, 2019. www.compassionfatigue.org/pages/symptoms.html.

Cooper, J.L., & F. Sogomonyan. 2010. "Trauma Faced by Children of Military Families: What Every Policymaker Should Know." National Center for Children in Poverty. www.nccp.org/publications/pdf/text_938.pdf.

COPPA (Children's Online Privacy Protection Rule of 1998). 2020. "Federal Trade Commission." www.ftc.gov/enforcement/rules/rulemaking-regulatory-reform-proceedings/childrens-online-privacy-protection-rule.

Copple, C., & S. Bredekamp, eds. 2009. *Developmentally Appropriate Practice in Early Childhood Programs Serving Children from Birth through Age 8*. 3rd ed. Washington, DC: NAEYC.

Council for Professional Recognition. 2019. "Asking the Question That Counts: Educators and Early Childhood Trauma." November 21. Washington, DC. www.cdacouncil.org/storage/documents/Media_Room/Asking_the_Question_that_Counts_Final.pdf.

Craig, S.E. 2008. *Reaching and Teaching Children Who Hurt*. Baltimore, MD: Brookes.

Craig, S.E. 2016. "The Trauma-Sensitive Teacher." *Educational Leadership* 74 (1): 28–32. www.ascd.org/publications/educational_leadership/sept16/vol74/num01/The_Trauma-Sensitive_Teacher.aspx.

Crecco, J. n.d. "Trauma Sensitivity During the IEP Process." *Federation for Children with Special Needs*. Accessed May 23, 2019. https://fcsn.org/rtsc/wp-content/uploads/sites/2/2013/11/Trauma-Sensitivity-During-the-IEP-Process.pdf.

DMDC (Defense Manpower Data Center). 2019. "DoD Personnel, Workforce Reports & Publications." www.dmdc.osd.mil/appj/dwp/dwp_reports.jsp.

Derhally, L.A. 2016. "The Importance of Childhood Friendships, and How to Nurture Them." *The Washington Post*, July 25. www.washingtonpost.com/news/parenting/wp/2016/07/25/the-importance-of-childhood-friendships-and-how-to-nurture-them.

Dionne-Dostie, E., N. Paquette, M. Lassonde, & A. Gallagher. 2015. "Multisensory Integration and Child Neurodevelopment." *Brain Science* 5 (1): 32–57. www.ncbi.nlm.nih.gov/pmc/articles/PMC4390790.

Dorado, J., & V. Zakrzewski. 2013. "How to Help a Traumatized Child in the Classroom." *Greater Good Magazine*, October 23. https://greatergood.berkeley.edu/article/item/the_silent_epidemic_in_our_classrooms.

Doran, G.T. 1981. "There's a S.M.A.R.T. Way to Write Management's Goals and Objectives." *Management Review* 70 (11): 35–36.

Dotson, L. 2017. "The Transformative Power of Trauma-Informed Teaching." *EdWeek,* November 21. www.edweek.org/tm/articles/2017/11/22/the-transformative-power-of-trauma-informed-teaching.html.

Downing, K. 2016. *Trauma Training Facilitator's Tool Kit.* Communities in Schools: Central Texas. https://ciscentraltexas.org/wp-content/uploads/2017/06/Trauma-Training-Toolkit-8-29-2016.pdf.

Eklund, K., & E. Rossen. 2016. "Guidance for Trauma Screening in Schools." *Defending Childhood State Policy Initiative,* September. www.nasponline.org/assets/Documents/Resources%20and%20Publications/Resources/Crisis/Guidance%20for%20Trauma%20Screening%20in%20Schools.pdf.

Epstein, R., & T. Gonzalez. n.d. *Gender & Trauma: Somatic Interventions for Girls in Juvenile Justice: Implications for Policy and Practice.* Georgetown Law Center on Poverty and Inequality. Accessed September 1, 2019. www.law.georgetown.edu/poverty-inequality-center/wp-content/uploads/sites/14/2017/08/gender-and-trauma-1.pdf.

Eschleman, K.J., J. Madsen, G. Alarcon, & A. Barelka. 2014. "Benefiting from Creative Activity: The Positive Relationships Between Creative Activity, Recovery Experiences, and Performance-Related Outcomes." *Journal of Occupational and Organizational Psychology* 87 (3): 579–98. https://doi.org/10.1111/joop.12064.

Everytown for Gun Safety. n.d. "Gun Safety in America." Accessed May 6, 2019. www.everytownresearch.org.

Felitti, V.J., R.F. Anda, D. Nordenberg, D.F. Williamson, A.M. Spitz, V. Edwards, M.P. Koss, & J.S. Marks. 1998. "Relationship of Childhood Abuse and Household Dysfunction to Many of the Leading Causes of Death in Adults: The Adverse Childhood Experiences (ACE) Study." *American Journal of Preventive Medicine* (14) 4: 245–58.

Ferlazzo, L. 2012. "Response: The Difference Between Parent 'Involvement' and Parent 'Engagement.' Q&A with Larry Ferlazzo." *Education Week* (blog), March 27. https://blogs.edweek.org/teachers/classroom_qa_with_larry_ferlazzo/2012/03/response_the_difference_between_parent_involvement_parent_engagement.html.

Fletcher, K.E. 2003. "Childhood Posttraumatic Stress Disorder." In *Child Psychopathology*, 2nd ed., eds. E.J. Mash & R.A. Barkley, 330–71. New York: Guilford Press.

Foran, L.M. 2009. "Listening to Music: Helping Children Regulate Their Emotions and Improve Learning in the Classroom." https://files.eric.ed.gov/fulltext/EJ868339.pdf.

Foster, J.D., G.P. Kuperminc, & A.W. Price. 2004. "Gender Differences in Posttraumatic Stress and Related Symptoms Among Inner-City Minority Youth Exposed to Community Violence." *Journal of Youth and Adolescence* 33 (1): 59–69.

Foundation for a Mindful Society. 2019. "Getting Started with Mindfulness." www.mindful.org/meditation/mindfulness-getting-started.

Freudenberger, H.J., & G. Richelson. 1980. *Burnout: The High Cost of High Achievement.* Norwell, MA: Anchor Press.

Friedman, S., & A. Mwenelupembe, eds. 2020. *Each & Every Child: Teaching Preschool with an Equity Lens.* Washington, DC: NAEYC.

Gaffrey, M.S., D.M. Barch, J. Singer, R. Shenoy, & J. L. Luby. 2013. "Disrupted Amygdala Reactivity in Depressed 4- to 6-Year-Old Children." *Journal of the American Academy of Child & Adolescent Psychiatry* 52 (7): 737–46.

Gaskill, R.L., & B.D. Perry. 2014. "The Neurological Power of Play." In *Creative Arts and Play Therapy for Attachment Problems*, eds. C.A. Malchiodi & D.A. Crenshaw, 178–96. New York: Guilford Press.

Gilliam, W.S. 2005. *Prekindergarteners Left Behind: Expulsion Rates in State Prekindergarten Systems.* New Haven, CT: Edward Zigler Center in Child Development and Social Policy. https://medicine.yale.edu/childstudy/zigler/publications/National%20Prek%20Study_expulsion_34774_284_5379_v1.pdf.

Gilliam, W.S., A.N. Maupin, C.R. Reyes, M. Accavitti & F. Shic. 2016. "Do Early Educators' Implicit Biases Regarding Sex and Race Relate to Behavior Expectations and Recommendations of Preschool Expulsions and Suspensions?" Research Study Brief. Yale Child Study Center, September 28. https://medicine.yale.edu/childstudy/zigler/publications/Preschool%20Implicit%20Bias%20Policy%20Brief_final_9_26_276766_5379_v1.pdf.

Ginwright, S. 2018. "The Future of Healing: Shifting from Trauma Informed Care to Healing Centered Engagement." May 31. https://medium.com/@ginwright /the-future-of-healing-shifting-from-trauma-informed -care-to-healing-centered-engagement-634f557ce69c.

Gladstone, M. 2014. "Gun/Weapon Play in Early Childhood." *The Children's Community School Blog,* December 17. https://childrenscommunity.wordpress .com/2014/12/17/gunweapon-play-in-early-childhood.

Gleiser, M. 2018. "Suffering from Nature Deficit Disorder? Try Forest Bathing." *NPR,* April 4. www.npr.org/sections /13.7/2018/04/04/599135342/suffering-from-nature -deficit-disorder-try-forest-bathing.

Gorski, P. 2008. "The Myth of the Culture of Poverty." *Educational Leadership* 65 (7): 32–36.

Government of Western Australia. n.d. "Child Development and Trauma Guide." Accessed June 1, 2019. www.dcp .wa.gov.au/ChildProtection/ChildAbuseAndNeglect /Documents/ChildDevelopmentAndTraumaGuide.pdf.

Green, J. 2011. "Research Shows Nature Helps with Stress." *The Dirt,* September 8. https://dirt.asla.org/2011/09/08 /research-shows-nature-helps-with-stress.

Greenberg, M. 2017. "Five Ways Mindfulness Makes Your Relationship Happier." *Psychology Today,* June 30. www.psychologytoday.com/us/blog/the-mindful-self -express/201706/five-ways-mindfulness-makes-your -relationship-happier.

Grise-Owens, E. 2019. "Self-Care A-Z: Self-Care Is Much More Than a Mask." *The New Social Worker.* www.socialworker.com/feature-articles/self-care/self -care-a-z-self-care-is-much-more-than-a-mask.

Grogan, J. 2013. "The Myth of Resilient Children." *Psychology Today,* February 15. www.psychologytoday .com/us/blog/encountering-america/201302/the-myth -resilient-children.

Gunn, J. n.d. "Self-Care for Teachers of Traumatized Students." *Resilient Educator,* Accessed September 1, 2019. https://education.cu-portland.edu/blog/classroom -resources/self-care-for-teachers.

Halgunseth, L.C., A. Peterson, D.R. Stark, & S. Moodie. 2009. *Family Engagement, Diverse Families, and Early Childhood Education Programs: An Integrated Review of the Literature.* Washington, DC: NAEYC & Pre-K Now. http://nieer.org/wp-content/uploads/2011/09/EDF _Literature20Review.pdf.

Hall, D.K., & J. Pearson. 2004. *Introducing Thinking Skills to Promote Resilience in Young Children. Reaching IN . . . Reaching OUT (RIRO).* Toronto, ON: Child & Family Partnership.

Hassinger-Das, B., K. Hirsh-Pasek, & R. Golinkoff. 2017. "The Case of Brain Science and Guided Play: A Developing Story." *Young Children* 72 (2): 45–50. www.naeyc.org/resources/pubs/yc/may2017/case -brain-science-guided-play.

Haughey, D. 2014. "A Brief History of SMART Goals." Project Smart, December 13. https://www.projectsmart .co.uk/brief-history-of-smart-goals.php

Henrich, C., & D. Gadaire. 2008. "Head Start and Parent Involvement." *Infants and Young Children* 21 (1): 56–69.

HHS (US Department of Health and Human Services) & ED (US Department of Education). 2016. "Policy Statement on Family Engagement: From the Early Years to the Early Grades." May 5. www2.ed.gov/about/inits /ed/earlylearning/files/policy-statement-on-family -engagement.pdf.

Himelstein, S. n.d. "9 Guidelines for Teaching Trauma-Informed Mindfulness to Teens." Center for Adolescent Studies. Accessed July 20, 2019. https:// centerforadolescentstudies.com/trauma-informed -mindfulness-with-teenagers-9-guidelines.

Hirsh-Pasek, K., R.M. Golinkoff, L.E. Berk, & D.G. Singer. 2009. *A Mandate for Playful Learning in Preschool: Presenting the Evidence.* New York: Oxford University Press.

Hopper, E.K., E.L. Bassuk, & J. Olivet. 2010. "Shelter from the Storm: Trauma-Informed Care in Homeless Service Settings." *The Open Health Services and Policy Journal* (2): 80–100.

Hudnall Stamm, B. 2009. "Professional Quality of Life: Compassion Satisfaction and Fatigue Version 5" (ProQOL). https://socialwork.buffalo.edu/content/dam /socialwork/home/self-care-kit/compassion-satisfaction -and-fatigue-stamm-2009.pdf.

Hughes, M., & W. Tucker. 2018. "Poverty as an Adverse Childhood Experience." *North Carolina Medical Journal* 79 (2): 124–26.

Integrated Learning Strategies. 2017. "BRAIN GYM: Simple Brain Gym Exercises to Awaken the Brain for Learning Readiness." January 19. https://ilslearningcorner.com /2017-01-brain-gym-simple-brain-gym-exercises-to -awaken-the-brain-for-learning-readiness.

James, T., & J. Countryman. 2012. "Psychiatric Effects of Military Deployment on Children and Families." *Innovations in Clinical Neuroscience* 9 (2): 16–20. www.ncbi.nlm.nih.gov/pmc/articles/PMC3312898.

Jennings, P.A. 2019a. "How to Help Students Dealing with Adversity." *Greater Good Magazine,* January 17. UC Berkeley. https://greatergood.berkeley.edu/article/item /how_to_help_students_dealing_with_adversity

Jennings, P.A. 2019b. "Teaching in a Trauma-Sensitive Classroom." *American Educator* 43 (2): 12–13.

Jensen, E. 2016. *Poor Students, Rich Teaching: Mindsets for Change.* Bloomington: IN: Solution Tree Press.

Johns Hopkins University. n.d. "Unintentional Injury Statistics." Accessed August 30, 2019. www .hopkinsmedicine.org/health/wellness-and-prevention /unintentional-injury-statistics.

Joseph, G.E., & P.S. Strain. 2004. "Building Positive Relationships with Young Children." *Young Exceptional Children* 7 (4): 21–23.

Joseph, G.E., & P.S. Strain. 2010. "Building Positive Relationships with Young Children." Preschool Training Modules, Module 1: "Promoting Children's Success: Building Relationships and Creating Supportive Environments." CSEFEL. http://csefel.vanderbilt.edu /modules/module1/handout5.pdf.

Klinic Community Health Centre. 2013. *Trauma-Informed: The Trauma Toolkit.* 2nd ed. http://trauma-informed .ca/wp-content/uploads/2013/10/Trauma-informed _Toolkit.pdf.

Koralek, D., K. Nemeth, & K. Ramsey. 2019. *Families & Educators Together: Building Great Relationships that Support Young Children.* Washington, DC: NAEYC.

Kuschner, D. 2012. "Play Is Natural to Childhood But School Is Not: The Problem of Integrating Play Into the Curriculum." *International Journal of Play* 1 (3): 242–49.

La Vigne, N.G., E. Davies, & D. Brazzell. 2008. "Broken Bonds: Understanding and Addressing the Needs of Children with Incarcerated Parents." Urban Institute, February 12. www.urban.org/research/publication /broken-bonds-understanding-and-addressing-needs -children-incarcerated-parents.

Ladson-Billings, G. 2011. "Boyz to Men? Teaching to Restore Black Boys' Childhood." *Race Ethnicity and Education* 14 (1): 7–15.

Lander, J. 2018. "Helping Teachers Manage the Weight of Trauma." Harvard Graduate School of Education, September 26. www.gse.harvard.edu/news/uk/18/09 /helping-teachers-manage-weight-trauma.

Lazar, K. 2019. "Positive Relationships Can Buffer Childhood Trauma and Toxic Stress, Researchers Say." *Boston Globe,* October 15. www.bostonglobe.com /metro/2019/10/15/positive-relationships-can-buffer -childhood-trauma-and-toxic-stress-researchers-say /ebR0F2XGqruN6ysJsMz9XO/story.html.

Lewis, K.R. 2015. "What If Everything You Knew About Disciplining Kids Was Wrong?" *Mother Jones,* July/ August. www.motherjones.com/politics/2015/07/schools -behavior-discipline-collaborative-proactive-solutions -ross-greene.

L!fe Solutions Counseling. 2018. "The Power of Gratitude." October 23. https://lifesolutions.io/gratitude-can-heal -trauma-and-change-your-life.

Livni, E. 2019. "There Is a Word for the Trauma Caused by Distance from Nature." February 24. https://qz.com /1557308/psychoterratica-is-the-trauma-caused-by -distance-from-nature.

Malik, R. 2017. "New Data Reveal 250 Preschoolers Are Suspended or Expelled Every Day." Center for American Progress, November 6. www.americanprogress.org /issues/early-childhood/news/2017/11/06/442280 /new-data-reveal-250-preschoolers-suspended-expelled -every-day.

Manitoba Trauma Information & Education Centre. n.d. a. "Mindfulness." Accessed January 16, 2020. http://trauma-recovery.ca/recovery/mindfulness.

Manitoba Trauma Information & Education Centre. n.d. b. "Mindfulness/MBSR." Accessed January 16, 2020. https://trauma-informed.ca/trauma-recovery /mindfulnessmbsr.

Mardell, B., D. Wilson, J. Ryan, K. Ertel, M. Krechevsky, & M. Baker. 2016. "Towards a Pedagogy of Play." Working paper. Project Zero. http://pz.harvard.edu/sites/default /files/Towards%20a%20Pedagogy%20of%20Play.pdf.

The Maryland Family Engagement Coalition. 2016. *The Early Childhood Family Engagement Framework Toolkit.* Baltimore, MD: Maryland State Department of Education. http://ascend.aspeninstitute.org/legacy /resources/MD%20family%20engagement%20toolkit.pdf.

Mayo Clinic. 2017. "Being Assertive: Reduce Stress, Communicate Better." May 9. www.mayoclinic.org /healthy-lifestyle/stress-management/in-depth /assertive/art-20044644.

Mayo Clinic. 2018. "Post-Traumatic Stress Disorder (PTSD)." www.mayoclinic.org/diseases-conditions /post-traumatic-stress-disorder/symptoms-causes /syc-20355967.

McNally, S., & R. Slutsky. 2018. "Teacher–Child Relationships Make All the Difference: Constructing Quality Interactions in Early Childhood Settings." *Early Child Development and Care* 188 (5): 508–23. https://doi.org/10.1080/03004430.2017.1417854.

Meeker, E. 2015. "Using Trauma-Sensitive Strategies to Support Family Engagement and Effective Collaboration. Transcript." Webinar. CADRE, December 3. www .cadreworks.org/resources/cadre-materials/using -trauma-sensitive-strategies-support-family-engagement -and-effective.

Menschner, C., & A. Maul. 2016. "Key Ingredients for Successful Trauma-Informed Care Implementation." Issue brief. Center for Health Care Strategies, Robert Wood Johnson Foundation, April. www.chcs.org/media /ATC_whitepaper_040616.pdf.

Meyers, L. 2014. "The Toll of Childhood Trauma." Issue brief. *Counseling Today,* June 23. https://ct.counseling .org/2014/06/the-toll-of-childhood-trauma.

Miller, C. 2014. "How Trauma Can Be Misdiagnosed as ADHD." Child Mind Institute, July 7. https://childmind .org/blog/how-trauma-can-be-misdiagnosed-as-adhd.

Miller, C. n.d. "How Trauma Affects Kids in School." Child Mind Institute. Accessed March 14, 2019. https:// childmind.org/article/how-trauma-affects-kids-school.

Milteer, R.M., & K.R. Ginsburg. 2011. "The Importance of Play in Promoting Healthy Child Development and Maintaining Strong Parent-Child Bond: Focus On Children in Poverty." *Pediatrics* 129 (1): e204–e213. https://pediatrics.aappublications.org/content/129 /1/e204.

MindTools. n.d. "SMART Goals." Accessed February 5, 2020. https://www.mindtools.com/pages/article/smart -goals.htm.

Moments for "Me." 2017. "Why Are Hobbies a Self Care Activity?" March 18. www.momentsformeonline.com /why-are-hobbies-a-self-care-activity.

Mwenelupembe, A. 2020. "6x. What You Can Do to Prevent Preschool Expulsion." *Teaching Young Children* 13 (3): 10–11.

NAEYC. 2009. "Developmentally Appropriate Practice in Early Childhood Programs Serving Children from Birth through Age 8." Position statement. Washington, DC: NAEYC. www.naeyc.org/positionstatements/dap.

NAEYC. 2018. *NAEYC Early Learning Program Accreditation Standards and Assessment Items.* Washington, DC: NAEYC. https://www.naeyc.org /sites/default/files/globally-shared/downloads /PDFs/accreditation/early-learning/standards_and _assessment_web_1.pdf.

NAEYC. 2019. "Advancing Equity in Early Childhood Education." Position statement. Washington, DC: NAEYC. www.naeyc.org/resources/position-statements/equity.

NAEYC. 2020. "Professional Standards and Competencies for Early Childhood Educators." Position statement. Washington, DC: NAEYC. www.naeyc.org/sites/default/files/globally-shared/downloads/PDFs/resources/position-statements/professional_standards_and_competencies_for_early_childhood_educators.pdf.

National Center on Safe Supportive Learning Environments. n.d. "Building Trauma-Sensitive Schools Handout Packet." Accessed February 28, 2019. https://safesupportivelearning.ed.gov/sites/default/files/Building_TSS_Handout_Packet_ALL.pdf.

National Resource Center on Children & Families of the Incarcerated. 2014. "Children and Families of the Incarcerated Fact Sheet." Rutgers University. https://nrccfi.camden.rutgers.edu/files/nrccfi-fact-sheet-2014.pdf.

Nature at the Confluence. n.d. "Let the Trees Heal: Shinrin Yoku (Forest Therapy)." Accessed October 24, 2019. https://natureattheconfluence.com/let-the-trees-heal-shinrin-yoku-forest-therapy.

NCCD Center for Girls and Young Women. n.d. "Understanding Trauma Through a Gender Lens." Accessed January 23, 2020. www.nccdglobal.org/sites/default/files/publication_pdf/understanding-trauma.pdf.

NCTSN (National Child Traumatic Stress Network). 2008a. "Child Trauma Toolkit for Educators." www.nctsn.org/resources/child-trauma-toolkit-educators.

NCTSN. 2008b. "Psychological and Behavioral Impact of Trauma: Elementary School Students." www.isbe.net/Documents/trauma-elementary.pdf.

NCTSN. 2010. "Stigma Surrounding Trauma Treatment in the Hispanic Community and Recommendations for Engagement in TF-CBT Treatment." Webinar. https://learn.nctsn.org/enrol/index.php?id=345.

NCTSN. 2011. "Secondary Traumatic Stress: A Fact Sheet for Child-Serving Professionals." www.nctsn.org/sites/default/files/resources/fact-sheet/secondary_traumatic_stress_child_serving_professionals.pdf.

NCTSN. 2013. *Child Welfare Trauma Training Toolkit*. www.nctsn.org/resources/child-welfare-trauma-training-toolkit.

NCTSN. 2016. "Spotlight on Culture: At Intersection of Trauma and Disabilities: A New Toolkit for Providers." Fact sheet. Spring. www.nctsn.org/sites/default/files/resources//spotlight_on_culture_intersection_of_trauma_and_disabilities_new_toolkit_for_providers.pdf.

NCTSN. 2017. "Addressing Race and Trauma in the Classroom: A Resource for Educators." www.nctsn.org/resources/addressing-race-and-trauma-classroom-resource-educators.

NCTSN. n.d. a. "About Child Trauma. What Is a Traumatic Event?" Accessed April 6, 2018. https://www.nctsn.org/what-is-child-trauma/about-child-trauma.

NCTSN. n.d. b. "Complex Trauma. Effects." Accessed April 6, 2018. www.nctsn.org/what-is-child-trauma/trauma-types/complex-trauma/effects.

NCTSN. n.d. c. "Sexual Abuse. Effects." Accessed April 8, 2018. www.nctsn.org/what-is-child-trauma/trauma-types/sexual-abuse/effects.

NCTSN. n.d. d. "Traumatic Grief. Trauma Types." Accessed April 6, 2018. www.nctsn.org/what-is-child-trauma/trauma-types/traumatic-grief.

NEA (National Education Association). 2016. *Teaching Children from Poverty and Trauma*. Washington, DC: NEA.

Nemeth, K., & P. Brillante. 2011. "Solving the Puzzle: Dual Language Learners with Challenging Behaviors." *Young Children* 66 (4): 12–17.

Nicholson, J., P.S. Driscoll, J. Kurtz, D. Márquez, & L. Wesley. 2020. *Culturally Responsive Self-Care Practices for Early Childhood Educators*. New York: Routledge.

Nicholson, J., L. Perez, & J. Kurtz. 2019. *Trauma-Informed Practices for Early Childhood Educators*. New York: Routledge.

NPR. 2015. "How Does Play Shape Our Development?" TED Radio Hour, March 27. www.npr.org/2015/03/27/395065944/how-does-play-shape-our-development.

Office of Justice Programs. n.d. Accessed August 21, 2019. "The Vicarious Trauma Toolkit. What Is Vicarious Trauma?" https://vtt.ovc.ojp.gov/about-the-toolkit.

Ollison, J. 2019. "Improving Teacher Retention by Addressing Teachers' Compassion Fatigue." PhD diss., University of the Pacific. https://scholarlycommons .pacific.edu/uop_etds/3602.

Ortiz R., & E.M. Sibinga. 2017. "The Role of Mindfulness in Reducing the Adverse Effects of Childhood Stress and Trauma." *Children* 4 (3): 16. www.ncbi.nlm.nih.gov/pmc /articles/PMC5368427.

Owens, J., & S.S. McLanahan. 2019. "Unpacking the Drivers of Racial Disparities in School Suspension and Expulsion." *Social Forces,* June 20. https://academic .oup.com/sf/advance-article/doi/10.1093/sf/soz095 /5521044.

Pearson, J., & D.K. Hall. 2017. *RIRO Resiliency Guidebook. Reaching Out . . . Reaching In.* Toronto, ON: First Folio Research Group.

Perry, B.D., & M. Szalavitz. 2017. *The Boy Who Was Raised as a Dog: And Other Stories From a Child Psychiatrist's Notebook—What Traumatized Children Can Teach Us About Loss, Love, and Healing.* Revised and updated ed. New York: Basic Books.

Peterson, K. 2016. "Helping Children Who Have Experienced Trauma to Make Friends." KITS (Kids In Transition to School), February 29. www .kidsintransitiontoschool.org/helping-children-who-have -experienced-trauma-to-make-friends.

Pevzner, H. 2014. "Is War Play Bad for Kids? The Surprising Truth: No. Learn Why Aggressive Play Helps Kids Become Compassionate Adults." *Scholastic Parents,* April 14. www.scholastic.com/parents/family-life/parent -child/war-play-bad-kids.html.

Pianta, R.C. 2001. *Student-Teacher Relationship Scale: Professional Manual.* Odessa, FL: Psychological Assessment Resources.

Presidential Task Force on Posttraumatic Stress Disorder and Trauma in Children and Adolescents. 2008. *Children and Trauma. Update for Mental Health Professionals.* Washington, DC: American Psychological Association. www.apa.org/pi/families/resources/children-trauma -update.aspx.

Preston, A. 2016. "In Defense of Hobbies. If You Want to Be a Better Person, Find Something to Do Outside of Work." June 12. https://qz.com/689526/hobbies-and-the -meaning-of-life.

Price, C. 2018. "Circle Preschool Program, A Best-Practices Model for Trauma-Informed Early Education." Voices for Virginia's Children, June 29. https://vakids.org/our -news/blog/circle-preschool-program-a-best-practices -model-for-trauma-informed-early-education.

Quitangon, G. 2019. "Vicarious Trauma in Clinicians: Fostering Resilience and Preventing Burnout." MJH Life Sciences, July 26. www.psychiatrictimes.com/burnout /vicarious-trauma-clinicians-fostering-resilience-and -preventing-burnout.

Raghavan, S.S., & P. Sandanapitchai. 2019. "Cultural Predictors of Resilience in a Multinational Sample of Trauma Survivors." *Frontiers in Psychology,* February 5. www.frontiersin.org/articles/10.3389/fpsyg.2019.00131 /full.

Rao, N., & K.J. Kemper. 2017. "Online Training in Specific Meditation Practices Improves Gratitude, Well-Being, Self-Compassion, and Confidence in Providing Compassionate Care Among Health Professionals." *The Journal of Evidence-Based Integrative Medicine* 22 (2): 237–41.

Reivich, K., & A. Shatté. 2002. *The Resilience Factor: 7 Keys to Finding Your Inner Strength and Overcoming Life's Hurdles.* New York: Broadway Books.

Reskin, B. 2012. "The Race Discrimination System." *Annual Review of Sociology* 38 (1): 17–35.

Resler, M. 2019. "Systems of Trauma: Racial Trauma." *Family & Children's Trust of Virginia.* www.fact.virginia .gov/wp-content/uploads/2019/05/Racial-Trauma -Issue-Brief.pdf.

Reynolds, G. 2015. "How Walking in Nature Changes the Brain." *The New York Times,* July 22. https://well.blogs .nytimes.com/2015/07/22/how-nature-changes-the -brain.

Rickard, C.L. 2018. "Self-Care and the Art of Saying 'No.'" Hope to Cope, May 7. www.hopetocope.com/depression -the-art-of-saying-no.

Roberts, A.L., S.E. Gilman, J. Breslau, N. Breslau, & K.C. Koenen. 2011. "Race/Ethnic Differences in Exposure to Traumatic Events, Development of Post-Traumatic Stress Disorder, and Treatment-seeking for Post-traumatic Stress Disorder in the United States." *Psychological Medicine* 41 (1): 71–83. www.ncbi.nlm.nih.gov/pmc /articles/PMC3097040.

Rossen, E. 2018. "Creating Trauma-Informed Individualized Education Programs: Integration of ACEs Into the Development of IEPs for Students through Grade 12." *CYF News,* November. www.apa.org/pi/families/resources /newsletter/2018/11/trauma-teaching.

Rotshtein, P., & I. Mitchell. 2018. "A Brief Introduction to Neuroscience." In *The Wiley Blackwell Handbook of Forensic Neuroscience,* eds. A.R. Beech, A.J. Carter, R.E. Mann, & P. Rotshtein, 25–58. Hoboken, NJ: John Wiley & Sons.

Sacks, V., & D. Murphey. 2018. "The Prevalence of Adverse Childhood Experiences, Nationally, by State, and by Race or Ethnicity." *Child Trends,* February 20. www.childtrends.org/publications/prevalence-adverse -childhood-experiences-nationally-state-race-ethnicity.

SAMHSA (Substance Abuse and Mental Health Services Administration). 2014a. *SAMHSA's Concept of Trauma and Guidance for a Trauma-Informed Approach.* HHS Publication No. (SMA) 14-4884. https://store .samhsa.gov/product/SAMHSA-s-Concept-of-Trauma -and-Guidance-for-a-Trauma-Informed-Approach /SMA14-4884.

SAMHSA. 2014b. *Trauma-Informed Care in Behavioral Health Services.* Treatment Improvement Protocol (TIP) Series 57. HHS Publication No. (SMA) 13-4801. www.integration.samhsa.gov/clinical-practice/SAMSA _TIP_Trauma.pdf.

Schwartz, K. 2019. "Why Mindfulness and Trauma- Informed Teaching Don't Always Go Together." *KQED News, MindShift,* January 27. www.kqed.org/mindshift /52881/why-mindfulness-and-trauma-informed -teaching-dont-always-go-together?fbclid=IwAR3CIcMjw 8T3VHHjZ7HcxsKClFSnD5sJnNw1Yu_KIYIyJ1t8nQgq GlEpXPw.

Scott, E. 2019. "5 Self-Care Practices for Every Area of Your Life." Verywell Mind, July 25. www.verywellmind.com /self-care-strategies-overall-stress-reduction-3144729.

Seligman, M.E.P. 2005. *Learned Optimism: How to Change Your Mind and Your Life.* New York: Vintage Books.

Seligman, M.E.P. 2007. *The Optimistic Child: A Proven Program to Safeguard Children Against Depression and Build Lifelong Resilience.* Boston, MA: Mariner Books.

Semple, R.J., J. Lee, D. Rosa, & L.F. Miller. 2010. "A Randomized Trial of Mindfulness-Based Cognitive Therapy for Children: Promoting Mindful Attention to Enhance Social-Emotional Resiliency in Children." *Journal of Child and Family Studies* 19 (2): 218–29.

Sherer Law Offices. n.d. "What Is the Difference Between Foster Care and Guardianship?" Accessed February 12, 2020. https://shererlaw.com/difference-foster-care -guardianship.

Singer, D., R.M. Golinkoff, & K. Hirsh-Pasek, eds. 2006. *Play = Learning: How Play Motivates and Enhances Children's Cognitive and Social-Emotional Growth.* New York: Oxford University Press.

Singh, M. 2014. "Got a Hobby? Might Be a Smart Professional Move." Shots: Health News from NPR, April 17. www.npr.org/sections/health-shots/2014/04/17 /303769531/could-those-weekend-pottery-classes-help -you-get-promoted-at-work.

Singh, N.N., G.E. Lancioni, A.S.W. Winton, B.T. Karazsia, & J. Singh. 2013. "Mindfulness Training for Teachers Changes the Behavior of Their Preschool Students." *Research in Human Development* 10 (3): 211–33. www.tandfonline.com/doi/full/10.1080/15427609 .2013.818484?scroll=top&needAccess=true.

Skilled at Life. n.d. "Why Hobbies Are Important." Accessed February 10, 2020. www.skilledatlife.com/why-hobbies -are-important.

Sorrels, B. 2015. *Reaching and Teaching Children Exposed to Trauma.* Louisville, NC: Gryphon House.

Sporleder, J., & H.T. Forbes. 2016. *The Trauma-Informed School: A Step-By-Step Implementation Guide for Administrators and School Personnel.* Boulder, CO: Beyond Consequences Institute.

START (National Consortium for the Study of Terrorism and Responses to Terrorism). 2018. "Global Terrorism Database." www.start.umd.edu/gtd.

Statman-Weil, K. 2015. Creating Trauma-Sensitive Classrooms. *Young Children* 70 (2). www.naeyc.org /resources/pubs/yc/may2015/trauma-sensitive -classrooms.

Stevens, J. 2015. "Does Poverty Cause ACES? Or Do ACES Cause Poverty?" February 23. www.acesconnection.com /blog/does-poverty-cause-aces-or-do-aces-cause-poverty.

Sue, D.W., C.M. Capodilupo, G.C. Torino, J.M. Bucceri, A.M.B. Holder, K.L. Nadal, & M. Esquilin. 2007. "Racial Microaggressions in Everyday Life." *American Psychologist* 62 (4): 271–86. https://gim.uw.edu/sites /gim.uw.edu/files/fdp/Microagressions%20File.pdf.

Szilagy, M. 2014. "Guidance for Foster/Kinship Caregivers." American Academy of Pediatrics, Healthy Foster Care America. www.aap.org/en-us/Documents/hfca_guidance _foster_kinship_caregivers.pdf.

Tang, Y., B. Hölzel, & M.I. Posner. 2015. "The Neuroscience of Mindfulness Meditation." *Nature Reviews Neuroscience* 16 (4): 213–25.

Taylor, L. 2013. "How to Be Assertive Not Aggressive." *Psychology Today*, May 4. www.psychologytoday.com /us/blog/tame-your-terrible-office-tyrant/201305/how -be-assertiv-not-aggressive.

Tec Center. 2017. "Ten Technology in Early Childhood Policy Statements You Should Know." Erikson Institute, March 6. http://teccenter.erikson.edu/tec/ten-technology-in-early -childhood-policy-statements-you-should-know.

Texas Children's Hospital. 2019. "The Impact of Toxic Stress in Children." www.texaschildrens.org/blog/impact -toxic-stress-children.

Transitional Support. n.d. "Burnout vs. Compassion Fatigue." Accessed August 19, 2019. http://transitionalsupport .com.au/transitional-phase/compassion-fatigue-trauma.

Treleaven, D. 2018. "Trauma Is Always Political: Social Context in Trauma-Informed Practice." *Mindfulness*, June 1. www.eomega.org/article/trauma-is-always -political?source=EPromoPur.MIND.ws.

Treleaven, D. 2019. "Trauma-Sensitive Solutions Checklist." https://davidtreleaven.com/https://davidtreleaven.com /wp-content/uploads/2019/03/TSM-Solutions-Checklist -v3.pdf.

Trent, M., D.G. Dooley, & J. Dougé. 2019. "The Impact of Racism on Child and Adolescent Health." *Pediatrics* 144 (2). https://doi.org/10.1542/peds.2019-1765.

Tull, M. 2020. "How Journaling Can Help with PTSD." Verywell Mind, February 19. www.verywellmind.com /how-to-use-journaling-to-cope-with-ptsd-2797594.

Turner, B. 2019. "Teaching First-Graders About Microaggressions: The Small Moments Add Up." *Teaching Tolerance,* March 26. www.tolerance.org /magazine/teaching-firstgraders-about-microaggressions -the-small-moments-add-up.

UN OHCHR (United Nations Office of the High Commissioner for Human Rights). 1989. "Convention on the Rights of the Child." www.ohchr.org/en /professionalinterest/pages/crc.aspx.

US Department of Education Office for Civil Rights. 2014. "Data Snapshot: School Discipline." Civil Rights Data Collection. Issue Brief No. 1, March 21. https:// ocrdata.ed.gov/Downloads/CRDC-School-Discipline -Snapshot.pdf.

US Department of Veterans Affairs. 2019. "PTSD Basics." www.ptsd.va.gov/understand/what/ptsd_basics.asp.

Vasandani, S. 2015. "Creating Environments that Reduce Children's Stress." *Exchange* (November/December): 40–43. https://tkcalifornia.org/wp-content/uploads /2017/07/environments-that-reduce-stress.pdf.

Wamser-Nanney, R., K.E. Cherry, C. Campbell, & E. Trombetta. 2018. "Racial Differences in Children's Trauma Symptoms Following Complex Trauma Exposure." *Journal of Interpersonal Violence.* https://journals.sagepub.com/doi/abs/10.1177 /0886260518760019.

Washington, V., ed. 2017. *Essentials for Child Development Associates Working with Young Children.* 4th ed. Washington, DC: Council for Professional Recognition.

Weare, K. 2012. "Evidence for the Impact of Mindfulness on Children and Young People." The Mindfulness in Schools Project, April. https://mindfulnessinschools.org/wp -content/uploads/2013/02/MiSP-Research-Summary -2012.pdf.

Weiss, H.B., M. Caspe, & M.E. Lopez. 2006. *Family Involvement in Early Childhood Education.* Cambridge, MA: Harvard Family Research Project.

Welch, K., & A.A. Payne. 2010. "Racial Threat and Punitive School Discipline." *Social Problems* 57 (1): 25–48. https://doi.org/10.1525/sp.2010.57.1.25.

Wethington, H.R., R.A. Hahn, D.S. Fuqua-Whitley, T.A. Sipe, A.E. Crosby, R. L. Johnson, A.M. Liberman, E. Mościcki, L.N. Price, F.K. Tuma, G. Kalra, & S.K. Chattopadhyay. 2008. "The Effectiveness of Interventions to Reduce Psychological Harm from Traumatic Events Among Children and Adolescents: A Systematic Review." *American Journal of Preventive Medicine* 35 (3): 287–313.

Whitebread, D., P. Coltman, H. Jameson, & R. Lander. 2009. "Play, Cognition and Self-Regulation: What Exactly Are Children Learning When They Learn Through Play?" *Educational and Child Psychology* 26 (2): 40–52.

Williams, J.M. With K. Scherrer. 2017. *Trauma Toolkit: Tools to Support the Learning and Development of Students Experiencing Childhood and Adolescent Trauma.* Washington, DC: FirstBook. https://firstbook .org/blog/2019/06/27/educator-resource-the-first-book -trauma-toolkit.

Williams, M.T. 2015. "The Link Between Racism and PTSD." *Psychology Today,* September 6. www.psychologytoday.com/us/blog/culturally-speaking /201509/the-link-between-racism-and-ptsd.

Williams, R. 2019. "10 Spiritual Self-Care Tips You Need to Know." The Chopra Center, March 28. https://chopra.com /articles/10-spiritual-self-care-tips-you-need-to-know.

van Woerkom, M. 2019. "SEL Tip: Practice Gratitude as a Form of Self-Care." Morningside Center for Teaching Social Responsibility, March 12. www.morningsidecenter .org/teachable-moment/lessons/sel-tip-practice -gratitude-form-self-care.

Wolpow, R., M.M. Johnson, R. Hertel, & S.O. Kincaid. 2016. *The Heart of Learning and Teaching: Compassion, Resiliency and Academic Success.* Washington State Office of Superintendent of Public Instruction. www.k12 .wa.us/sites/default/files/public/compassionateschools /pubdocs/theheartoflearningandteaching.pdf.

Wright, B.L. 2020. "Black Boys Matter: Strategies for a Culturally Responsive Classroom." In *Each & Every Child: Teaching Preschool with an Equity Lens,* eds. S. Friedman & A. Mwenelupembe, 77–81. Washington, DC: NAEYC.

Wright, T. 2017. "Supporting Students Who Have Experienced Trauma." Talk presented at North American Montessori Teachers' Association conference, New Orleans LA, January 12–15, 2017. https://files.eric .ed.gov/fulltext/EJ1144506.pdf.

Yogman, M., A. Garner, J. Hutchinson, K. Hirsh-Pasek, & R.M. Golinkoff. 2018. "The Power of Play: A Pediatric Role in Enhancing Development in Young Children." *Pediatrics* 142 (3): 1–17. https://pediatrics .aappublications.org/content/142/3/e20182058.

Youth.gov. n.d. "Trauma." Accessed January 14, 2020. https://youth.gov/youth-topics/children-of-incarcerated -parents/children-who-have-experienced-trauma.

Zacarian, D., L. Alvarez-Ortiz, & J. Haynes. 2017a. *Teaching to Strengths: Supporting Students Living with Trauma, Violence, and Chronic Stress.* Alexandria, VA: ASCD.

Zacarian, D., L. Alvarez-Ortiz, & J. Haynes. 2017b. "Teaching to Strengths: Supporting Students Living with Trauma, Violence, and Chronic Stress." Webinar. ASCD, September 19. www.ascd.org/professional-development /webinars/teaching-to-strengths-webinar.aspx.

ZERO TO THREE. 2016. "Three Building Blocks of Reflective Supervision." March 8. www.zerotothree.org/resources /412-three-building-blocks-of-reflective-supervision.

Ziegler, E.H. 2011. "Researcher Finds Gender Differences in Child Trauma." *Center on Trauma and Children, University of Kentucky.* https://uknow.uky.edu/research /social-sciences/researcher-finds-gender-differences -child-trauma.

Zigler, E.F., D.G. Singer, & S.J. Bishop-Josef, eds. 2004. *Children's Play: The Roots of Reading.* Washington, DC: ZERO TO THREE.

Zosh, J.N., E.J. Hopkins, H. Jensen, C. Liu, D. Neale, K. Hirsh-Pasek, S.L. Solis, & D. Whitebread. 2017. *Learning Through Play: A Review of the Evidence.* Billund, Denmark: LEGO Foundation. www.legofoundation.com /media/1063/learning-through-play_web.pdf.

Index

A

ABCDE model, reframing negative thinking, 36–37, 105
acute trauma, 4
administrator support
   creating a TIC program, 90
   TIC, 86
adverse childhood experiences (ACEs),
     5–6, 8, 14, 16, 17, 27, 54, 60, 77
advocacy, 92
aggressive behaviors, sign of toxic stress, 23
anxiety, trauma and, 17
art
   music, and dance, 35
   supporting play in the center, 67
assault, 13
A Terrible Thing Happened (Holmes), 45
attention-deficit/hyperactivity disorder
     (ADHD), trauma and, 17
autism, trauma and, 17
automobile crashes, 12

B

Berman, Dr. Marc, 102
bibliotherapy, 44–46. 66. 87
*B is for Breathe: The ABCs of Coping with Fussy
    and Frustrating Feelings* (Boyd), 46
blocks, supporting play in the center, 65
blogs, 84
books
   for children with trauma experience, 44–46
   sample reading experience, 45
brain development
   circuits and connections, 19
   experience, brain connections and, 20
burnout, 96

C

calming center, 41, 44, 56, 82
celebrate joys of life, 38
Centers for Disease Control and Prevention
     (CDC), study on childhood trauma, 5–6
challenging behaviors, positive guidance, 32–33, 35
children
   connecting with, 50–60
   educators as a critical resource, 3

positive interactions with, 58–59
   relationships with peers, 53–54
   trauma effects on brains, 19–25
   trauma prevalence, 2
Children's Defense Fund, poverty definition, 8
Children's Online Privacy Protection Act (COPPA 2020), 84
Circle Preschool Program, 90
cognition and academic learning, trauma effects, 20
compassion fatigue, 5, 97
complex trauma, 4
connecting with children, 50–60
cooking, supporting play in the center, 67
culture
   effects on children's resilience, 29
   trauma and, 16

D

death and dying talk, sign of toxic stress, 24
deployment, 11
depression, trauma and, 17
development, trauma effects on, 22
developmentally appropriate practice (DAP), 4
differing influences, children's trauma experiences, 28–29
disability, trauma and, 17
discovery, supporting play in the center, 66
divorce or separation, ACE, 5
domestic violence, ACE, 5
Don't Feed the Worry Bug (Green), 46
Dotson, Lauren, 91
dramatic play, supporting play in the center, 65

E

eating pattern changes, sign of toxic stress, 2
educator–family meetings, 80–81
educators (teachers)
   advocacy, 92
   connecting with families, 79–84
   as a critical resource, 3
   partnering with families, 72–84
   print and digital resources for, 109–110
   supporting families in supporting children, 77–78
   training in trauma response, 1
   use of technology, 83–84
   video clips and webinars for, 110
   web resources for, 110

Acknowledgments

Writing a book is always a team effort. Many talented individuals kindly contributed to this one. We wish to thank the following:

> Shaelyn Amaio, whose artistry helped us convey our thoughts in pictures as well as words

> Dr. Casey Stockstill, whose expertise in Diversity, Equity, Accessibility, and Inclusion (DEAI) and young children kept us focused

> Ellen Galinsky for her thoughtful conversations in helping to shape the direction of the book, ensuring a focus on a healing-centered approach in which children are not defined by their trauma

> Karen Nemeth, Sally Durbin, and Dr. Linda Espinosa for their knowledge of how trauma affects children who speak a home language other than English

> Whit Hayslip for his expertise in special education and trauma's effects on children with disabilities

> Holly Bohart, senior editor at NAEYC, for her skills, knowledge, and graciousness in guiding us through the process of completing this book

About the Authors

Sarah Erdman is an experienced early childhood educator and museum professional. Her research and professional practice explore ways museums and educators can connect to make meaningful experiences for young children.

Sarah founded Cabinet of Curiosities LLC and has been an early childhood consultant for numerous museum and educational institutions. She publishes regularly through NAEYC and the American Alliance of Museums.

Sarah earned an MAT in Museum Education from The George Washington University and an AAS in Early Childhood Development from the Northern Virginia Community College. She currently teaches at FB Meekins Cooperative Preschool and is on the board of the Northern Virginia AEYC.

Laura J. Colker, EdD, is an author, lecturer, and trainer with 40 years of experience. She has written or contributed to over 150 publications, educational videos, and PBS programs.

Laura is most widely known as a coauthor of *The Creative Curriculum for Preschool,* now in its sixth edition. Her two most recent coauthored books are *High-Quality Early Childhood Programs: The What, Why, and How* and *Making Lemonade: Teaching Young Children How to Think Optimistically.*

For nine years Laura was a contributing editor to NAEYC's *Teaching Young Children.* She has also been a consultant to numerous education-related institutions and organizations and was a founder of the military's Sure Start program.

Elizabeth C. Winter, MD, is a psychiatrist living in Baltimore, Maryland. She is a senior physician with the Department of Veterans Affairs, Office of the Inspector General, and a faculty member of the Johns Hopkins Hospital Department of Psychiatry and Behavioral Sciences. Elizabeth began her career in private practice and became the co-director of the Johns Hopkins Anxiety Disorders Clinic. She later joined the faculty of University of Maryland before starting at the VA OIG in 2018.

Elizabeth has worked in medical education for more than 10 years and has published extensively on issues related to psychiatry. Elizabeth graduated from Johns Hopkins School of Medicine.

More NAEYC Books to Support Children & Families

Anti-Bias Education for Young Children and Ourselves
Second Edition by Louise Derman-Sparks, Julie Olsen Edwards, and Catherine M. Goins

More than ever, young children need educators who can help them navigate and thrive in a world of great diversity, educators who can give them and their families the tools to make the world a more fair place for themselves and for each other.

You can be that educator in children's lives. This classic resource, now expanded and updated, is your guide to building a strong anti-bias program, including learning to know yourself.

Whether you're new to anti-bias work or seasoned in it, you'll find inspiration and support here as you walk this journey and meet and work with other travelers.

Item 1143 • 2020 • 208 pages

Families and Educators Together:
Building Great Relationships that Support Young Children
by Derry Koralek, Karen N. Nemeth, and Kelly Ramsey

Home–school relationships have always been a cornerstone of children's success and well-being. Cultivating positive, supportive partnerships between educators and families, essential to this relationship, is an ongoing process, one that needs reciprocal respect and communication to nurture and grow. Use the strategies, resources, and information discussed in this book to develop and embed a culture of family engagement in all aspects of your early childhood program, from curriculum planning to addressing children's individual needs.

Item 1139 • 2019 • 140 pages

Spotlight on Young Children:
Social and Emotional Development by Rossella Procopio and Holly Bohart, Eds.

Children's experiences and relationships during their formative years have a far-reaching impact, and early childhood professionals play a critical role in fostering the social and emotional competence children need to process and learn from these interactions. Explore how teachers can use everyday opportunities to help children develop the social and emotional skills essential to their future well-being and success.

Item 2850 • 2017 • 116 pages

Ethics and the Early Childhood Educator
Third Edition by Stephanie Feeney and Nancy K. Freeman

The NAEYC Code of Ethical Conduct is an essential resource for every early childhood educator. This third edition of *Ethics and the Early Childhood Educator* shows you how to use the Code to guide your actions and responses to challenging situations in your work with children, their families, colleagues, and the community. Real cases from early childhood programs illustrate the process of identifying and addressing ethical dilemmas by applying the NAEYC Code.

Numerous reflection questions encourage you to think deeply about how your own experiences relate to the examples. The Code and this book are resources you can turn to again and again as you seek to make the right decisions for young children and their families.

Item 1134 • 2018 • 160 pages

Rituals and Traditions: Fostering a Sense of Community in Preschool

by Jacky Howell and Kimberly Reinhard

Rituals and traditions in preschool programs have the power to shape classroom routines into times that

> Build meaningful connections and bonds among children, families, and teachers

> Foster a sense of belonging

> Create a positive learning environment

The practical information and examples in this book answer the questions of why rituals and traditions are important and how teachers can incorporate them into their daily, weekly, monthly, and yearly plans to create a supportive, caring community.

Item 183 • 2015 • 128 pages

Discover NAEYC!

The National Association for the Education of Young Children (NAEYC) promotes high-quality early learning for all young children, birth through age 8, by connecting early childhood practice, policy, and research. We advance a diverse, dynamic early childhood profession and support all who care for, educate, and work on behalf of young children.

NAEYC members have access to award-winning publications, professional development, networking opportunities, professional liability insurance, and an array of members-only discounts.

Accreditation—NAEYC.org/accreditation

Across the country, **NAEYC Accreditation of Early Learning Programs** and **NAEYC Accreditation of Early Childhood Higher Education Programs** set the industry standards for quality in early childhood education. These systems use research-based standards to recognize excellence in the field of early childhood education.

Advocacy and Public Policy—NAEYC.org/policy

NAEYC is a leader in promoting and advocating for policies at the local, state, and federal levels that expand opportunities for all children to have equitable access to high-quality early learning. NAEYC is also dedicated to promoting policies that value early childhood educators and support their excellence.

Global Engagement—NAEYC.org/global

NAEYC's Global Engagement department works with governments and other large-scale systems to create guidelines to support early learning, as well as early childhood professionals throughout the world.

Professional Learning—NAEYC.org/ecp

NAEYC provides face-to-face training, technology-based learning, and Accreditation workshops—all leading to improvements in the knowledge, skills, and practices of early childhood professionals.

Publications and Resources—NAEYC.org/publications

NAEYC publishes some of the most valued resources for early childhood professionals, including award-winning books, *Teaching Young Children* magazine, and *Young Children*, the association's peer-reviewed journal. NAEYC publications focus on developmentally appropriate practice and enable members to stay up to date on current research and emerging trends, with information they can apply directly to their classroom practice.

Signature Events—NAEYC.org/events

NAEYC hosts three of the most important and well-attended annual events for educators, students, administrators, and advocates in the early learning community.

NAEYC's Annual Conference is the world's largest gathering of early childhood professionals.

NAEYC's Professional Learning Institute is the premier professional development conference for early childhood trainers, faculty members, researchers, systems administrators, and other professionals.

The **NAEYC Public Policy Forum** provides members with resources, training, and networking opportunities to build advocacy skills and relationships with policymakers on Capitol Hill.

NAEYC.org/membership